CASE
software
& books

NUTRITION FOCUSED PHYSICAL ASSESSMENT: MAKING CLINICAL CONNECTIONS

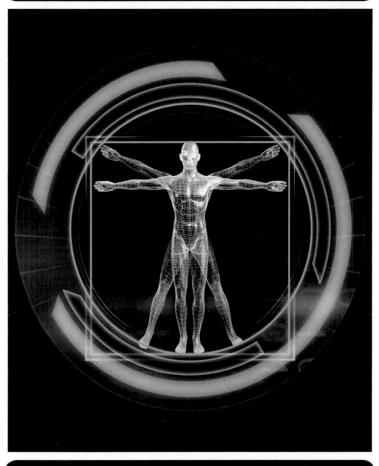

MARY D. LITCHFORD, PhD, RDN, LDN

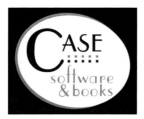

PREFACE

Nutrition Focused Physical Assessment (NFPA) has been part of the dietetics curriculum since the late 1990s, yet from my observation as a speaker and consultant, it is not an integral part of practice of all RDNs. Dietitians in Nutrition Support DPG have been trailblazers in this area producing a video entitled *Nutrition-Focused Physical Assessment Skills for Dietitians* in 1997.

In my clinical practice, I learned how to do nursing assessment for fluid accumulation, wound assessment and other chronic disease assessments in my first job. Those were invaluable skills that served as a foundation for doing NFPA of wounds. I built on these fundamental skills through collaborative work with nursing colleagues and continuing education. Over the years I have added other aspects of NFPA to my clinical practice. The delineation of components of NFPA outlined in the *International Dietetics and Nutrition Terminology Reference Manual (2009, 2011)* and the resurgent interest in defining characteristics of malnutrition by etiology has spurred my interest in speaking and writing on this topic.

Nutrition Focused Physical Assessment: Making Clinical Connections is the first edition. While it seemed like an exhaustive review in its production, medicine is constantly evolving. Please feel free to share with me ways in which you use NFPA in your clinical practice. My goal is to help practitioners move beyond their current level of expertise and gain a greater understanding of the cascade of events from diagnosis through treatment with positive outcomes.

Mary D. Litchford, PhD, RDN, LDN

ABOUT THE AUTHOR

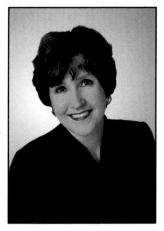

Dr. Mary Litchford, PhD, RDN, LDN is an acclaimed speaker, author, medical-legal expert and consultant to health care providers. She received her PhD in human nutrition from the University of North Carolina-Greensboro. Her professional career has included clinical practice in public health, home care, and long term care, university teaching and business consulting. She is president of CASE Software & Books, a professional and educational resource company. Dr. Litchford is well-known for her advanced level presentations, scholarly articles, textbook chapters and professional reference books on leading-edge clinical nutrition topics. She is a member of the Academy of Nutrition & Dietetics and serves as president of the National Pressure Ulcer Advisory Panel. Dr. Litchford has received numerous national awards for her contributions to the field of clinical nutrition.

Other advanced level reference books and CE courses to use in working with patients/residents include:

Laboratory Assessment of Nutritional Status: Bridging Theory & Practice (2017)

Nutrition & Pressure Injuries: Putting the New Guidelines into Practice (2016)

Common Denominators of Declining Nutritional Status (2013)

TABLE OF CONTENTS

LIST OF TABLES

LIST OF FIGURES & PHOTOGRAPHS

List of Figures & Photographs

List of Figures & Photographs

List of Figures & Photographs

List of Figures & Photographs

Chapter 1
Introduction & Objectives

Physical Examination vs. Nutrition Focused Physical Assessment: Overview

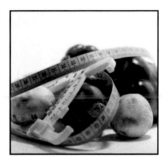

Traditionally physicians, nurses, nurse practitioners, and physician assistants were the primary medical team members who performed the health and physical (H&P) assessment. However, physical therapists, speech and language pathologists, occupational therapists and other allied health professionals perform portions of the overall physical assessment that is specific to their discipline. Nutrition-focused physical assessment (NFPA)was added to the dietetic curriculum in 1997! It follows to reason that RDNs should embrace a more hands-on approach to demonstrate our value to the medical team.

NFPA involves a hands-on assessment of the patient specific to nutrition-related components of health. The International Dietetics and Nutrition Terminology Reference Manual (2011) defines NFPA as:

findings from an evaluation of body systems, muscle and subcutaneous fat wasting, oral health, suck, swallow/breathe ability, appetite and affect.

NFPA is a focused assessment and does not replace the comprehensive history and physical exam performed by physicians and nurses. Use data from the comprehensive H&P exam to identify specific areas to include in the NFPA and to support nutrition diagnoses.

Legal Issues in NFPA

Is NFPA included in your 'scope of practice?' Scope of practice for licensed health care professionals is a state-based legislative function. Not all states have licensure for dietitians. Scope of practice dictates the range and type of activities a healthcare professional can legally perform and the responsibility and accountability of performance. For licensed dietitians, the state licensure law may outline your scope of practice in either general terms, more detailed terms or not at all. Since no two licensure statues are identical, it is the individual's responsibility to determine the legal requirements to practice in the states where services are provided. Lack of a state statute for dietitians does not eliminate professional responsibility or accountability. Your scope of practice may be delineated by your employer and supported by your continuing education plan. Also, other licensed healthcare professionals(i.e. nursing or pharmacy) may contain content that preclude other healthcare professions from performing or engaging in certain activities. The Academy's Quality Management Web site provides information and links to a variety of resources to assist the credentialed dietitian in determining requirements. http://www.eatright.org/quality/

Every RDN has an individual scope of practice as defined by the Scope of Dietetics Practice Framework. Every credentialed dietitian must be competent to do what he/she is doing in practice. Refer to the Scope of Dietetic Practice Framework, Standards of Practice (SOP) and Standards of Professional Performance (SOPP), and Academy's Code of Ethics for more information. http://www.eatright.org/ HealthProfessionals /content.aspx?id=6867. Selected

Dietetic Practice Groups (DPG) have focused SOP and SOPP available to members. Refer to other resources at the end of Chapter 1. The SOP that reflects the four steps in NCP are relevant to RDNs providing direct patient care. NFPA is part of the nutrition assessment step (Stieber, 2011). More details are included in Chapter 2.

Accountability & Responsibility

Every RDN is expected to practice only at the level at which he/she is competent (refer to Dietetics Career Development Guide.) Accreditation agencies focus surveys on practitioner competency and professional responsibility to provide safe, effective and quality care. RDNs are encouraged to pursue additional professional education and training to enhance their scope of practice and become advanced level practitioners.

RDNs who plan to incorporate hands-on NFPA must be able to demonstrate sufficient knowledge and skills appropriate to their care setting and job duties. Advanced level practitioners have expanded their scope of practice through professional education, hands-on training in clinical settings, speciality certifications and experience. As you embark on expanding your scope of practice to include NFPA, dedicate time and attention to acquiring more knowledge, find clinical settings to apply the new information under the guidance of a trained professional. Work collaboratively with advanced level practitioners or other health care team members to hone your skills in interpreting NFPA findings. Demonstrate NFPA skills using a competency-based format or as defined by your employer.

Utilize your Professional Development Portfolio to structure the pathway to attaining skills and competence in NFPA.

Professionals working in CMS funded healthcare facilities must follow the regulations specific to competency of technical personal. Refer to http://www.cms.gov for specific regulations governing your clinical setting.

Obstacles to NFPA

Why are RDNs resistant to doing NFPA? Obstacles may include limited training and experience in doing NFPA. Some feel more comfortable with a 'hands off' approach to nutrition assessment thus avoding the possibility of encroaching on the 'professional turf' of others. For some RDNs, changing the way an assessment is conducted is unsettling and appears to be time consuming. As RDNs embraced NCP, NFPA is simply another vital tool to demonstrate our expertise as the nutrition expert (Brand, 2010; Mackle, 2003; Stankorb, 2010).

In the last 30 years, RDNs have witnessed allied health care professionals adding responsibilities once unique to RDNs such as recommending consistency modified diets, determining fluid needs, tracking weight loss and making recommendations for liberalizing therapeutic diets or adding nutritional supplements. It is time to take hold of the unique components of the physical assessment specific to nutrition diagnoses. While RDNs can be trained to perform all components of a physical examination, most will work collaboratively with other medical team members and limit the assessment to those aspects that relate to nutrition concerns (Iannotta, 2010; Pieloch, 2010).

Purpose, Objectives & CE Options

Nutrition Focused Physical Assessment: Making Clinical Connections is sold as either a reference text or 14 CE Level III self-study course. The information is valuable for RDNs, nurses and other healthcare practitioners working with patients or residents in a variety of healthcare settings. The purpose of the course is to provide science based information which assists advanced level practitioners to develop skills in NFPA that support the nutrition diagnoses. NFPA also provides RDNs with objective tools to measure outcomes and demonstrate value to the medical team.

Reading a reference text and completing the CE course is the first step to enhancing your professional toolbox. The next step is to practice these skills in a supervised clinical setting. Work with your supervisor to establish competency based assessment tools to document mastery of specific aspects of NFPA. Collaborative assessment using NFPA is one way to expand your scope of practice and to demonstrate your value to the medical team.

Information for Self-Study Course Participants

For purchasers of the self-study course, either online case studies or a CD of case studies, is included for application of concepts. Each case study provides a medical profile of the patient/resident followed by a series of questions. Users receive specific, interactive assistance for any errors.

For the most effective use of the self-study course, users should have a clear understanding of medical nutrition therapy (MNT), interpreting abnormal patterns of medical data including all vital signs, laboratory values, medical physiology, common physiological changes that occur with injury, surgery or aging, disease processes and the physiology, common physiological changes that occur with injury, surgery or aging, disease processes and the relationship between changes in laboratory values, food-medication interactions and changes in general health.

Objectives

At the completion of this session the successful learner will be able to:

1. Explain the relationship between nutrition status indicators and changes in overall health.
2. Discuss NFPA as a component of Nutrition Care Process.
3. Describe the basic components of NFPA in terms of body systems and vital signs.
4. Describe normal appearance for skin, hair and nails.
5. Identify potential nutrient deficiencies associated with changes in skin, hair and nails using NFPA.
6. Identify signs of wound healing using NFPA.
7. Differentiate the three types of hydration dysregulation using NFPA.
8. Discuss criteria for assessing malnutrition using NFPA techniques.
9. Discuss techniques for assessing oral health and mastication.
10. Discuss techniques used to assess the digestive system.
11. Identify potential macronutrient deficiencies using NFPA.
12. Identify potential micronutrient deficiencies using NFPA.

CDR Learning Codes that can apply to this course include 3000, 3020, 3030, 3040, 3080, 5000, 5010, 5020, 5030, 5040, 5050, 5090, 5100, 5230, 5280, 5380 or other applicable codes.

Information for Self-Study Course Participants: Online Users

Your confirmation email includes the computer links to the online case studies and competency testing. These links expire in TEN DAYS! Be sure to bookmark these links for later use. If you are unable to access the URL links when it is time to complete the case studies or competency testing, please contact us by email or phone. We will resend the links promptly.

Once you have read the text, apply your knowledge with the online case studies. Users are asked to respond to a variety of questions. The case studies provide feedback to the correctness of your answer. Complete each case study and then take the online exam. You must score 70 percent on the competency exam to receive a Certificate of Completion. You may take the online exam more than once to achieve this benchmark. Once online users have passed the competency exam, please complete the Professional Continuing Education Survey and print your Certificate of Completion.

Hard Copy Users
Your order included a CD of case studies and a paper competency exam with answer sheet. Once you have read the text, apply your knowledge with the CD of case studies. Users are asked to respond to a variety of questions. The case studies provide feedback to the correctness of your answer. Complete each case study and then take the paper competency exam. You must score 70 percent on the competency exam to receive a Certificate of Completion. Please complete the Professional Continuing Education Survey and either mail or fax your answer sheet and survey to the address on the answer sheet. Keep a copy of your answer sheet and Professional Continuing Education Survey for your records. A Certificate of Completion will be mailed to you within 10 working days.

Please call or email us if you do not receive your Certificate of Completion within two weeks after it was mailed to CASE Software & Books. If you have a tight deadline to meet,

we will be happy to fax or email your Certificate of
Completion to you per your instructions.

Other Users

If you purchased this course from a source other than CASE
Software & Books, follow the instructions for completing the
self-study course provided at the time of your purchase.

Other Resources for Healthcare Professionals

Other vital reference books and CE courses to use in
working with patients/residents with wounds from CASE
Software & Books include:

*Laboratory Assessment of
Nutritional Status: Bridging Theory
& Practice* (2017)

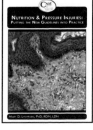

*Nutrition & Pressure Injuries: Putting
the New Guidelines into Practice*
(2016)

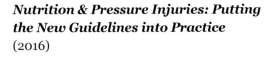

*Common Denominators of Declining
Nutritional Status*(2013)

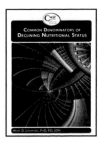

References:

American Dietetic Association (ADA). International dietetics & nutrition terminology reference manual. Chicago, IL: ADA, 2011.

ADA Quality Management Web site. Accessed October 2011 at: http://www.eatright.org/quality/.

Scope of Dietetics Practice Framework. American Dietetic Association Health Community. Accessed October 2011 at: http://www.eatright.org/HealthProfessionals /content.aspx?id=6867.

The Scope of Dietetics Practice Framework. Accessed October 2011 at: http://www.eatright.org/scope/.

ADA. Scope of Dietetics Practice Framework Definition of Terms. Accessed October 2011 at: http://www.eatright.org/scope/

ADA. Ethics opinion: dietetics professionals are ethically obligated to maintain personal competence in practice. *JADA*. 2003;103:633–635.

ADA/Commission on Dietetic Registration. Code of ethics for the profession of dietetics and process for consideration of ethics issues. *JADA*. 2009;109:1461–1467.

ADA Quality Management Committee. ADA revised 2008 standards of practice for registered dietitians in nutrition care; standards of professional performance for registered dietitians; standards of practice for dietetic technicians, registered, in nutrition care; and standards of professional performance for dietetic technicians, registered. *JADA*. 2008;108:1538–1542.e9.

ADA Practice Applications. Nutrition care process and model part I: the 2008 update. *JADA*. 2008:108:1113–1117.

Brand RM, Touger-Decker R, Radler Rigassio D, Parrott JS. Usage patterns of nutrition-focused physical assessment by the registered dietitian following completion of a nutrition-focused physical assessment program [abstract]. *JADA*. 2010;110(suppl):A–25.

Iannotta JA, Rigassio Radler D, Parrott JS. Nutrition focused physical examination practices of RD members of the oncology nutrition dietetic practice group and board certified specialists in oncology nutrition [abstract]. *JADA*. 2010;110(suppl):A–19.

Mackle TJ, Touger-Decker R, RD's use of physical assessment parameters in profession practice. *JADA*. 2003;103:1632–1637.

Pieloch D, Byham-Gray L, Brody R. A delphi study: using job functions to assist in defining levels of practice for dietitians practicing in nephrology care [abstract]. *JADA*. 2010;110(suppl):A–25.

Stankorb SM, Rigassio-Radler D, Nutrition-focused physical examination practices of registered dietitians. *Top Clin Nutr*. 2010;25:335–344.

Stieber,M Scope of practice and legal issues in nutrition-focused physical examination. *Support Line* April, 2011, 2-6.

Other Resources:
Focus Area Standards of Practice and Professional Performance: http://www.eatright.org/sop/
• Revised SOP and SOPP for RDs in Diabetes Care (January 2011 Journal article)
• SOP and SOPP for RDs in Oncology Nutrition Care (February 2010 Journal article)
• SOP and SOPP for RDs in Nephrology Care (September 2009 Journal article) • SOP and SOPP for RDs in Pediatric Nutrition (August 2009 Journal article)
• SOPP for RDs in Education of Dietetics Practitioners (April 2009 Journal article)
• SOP and SOPP for RDs in Sports Dietetics (March 2009 Journal article)
• SOPP for RDs in Management Food and Nutrition Systems (March 2009 Journal article)
• SOP and SOPP for RDs in Nutrition Support (October 2007 Journal article)
• SOP and SOPP for RDs in Behavioral Health Care (April 2006 Journal article)

Chapter 2
Getting Started

Nutrition Care Process

The Academy's Quality Management Committee appointed the Nutrition Care Model Workgroup to develop a new systematic process for RDNs to use in clinical practice. The NCP and model were published in 2003. Since then the Academy has published numerous resources for RDNs to transition their current practice to a standardized process for providing care. The NCP includes four steps:

- Nutrition assessment
- Nutrition diagnosis
- Nutrition intervention
- Nutrition monitoring and evaluation

Figure 2.1. Components of NCP

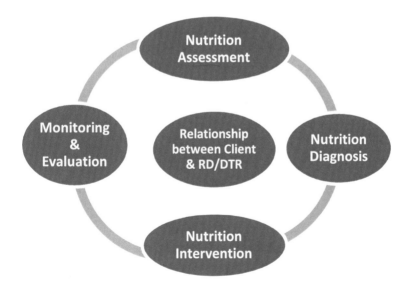

RDNs unfamiliar with NCP should refer to Academy's *International Dietetics & Nutrition Terminology Reference Manual* (2011) for more information.

NFPA is one of the components of nutrition care process under step 1, nutrition assessment. Information gathered in the NFPA is used in conjunction with food and nutrition history, lab and medical test results and client history to accurately identify one or more nutrition diagnosis(es). These five components give the RDN a global view of the nutrition-related issues and concerns.

In addition, nutrition-related physical characteristics associated with pathophysiological states are derived from:
- interview
- medical record
- collaboration with other healthcare team members

Figure 2.2. Components of Nutrition Assessment

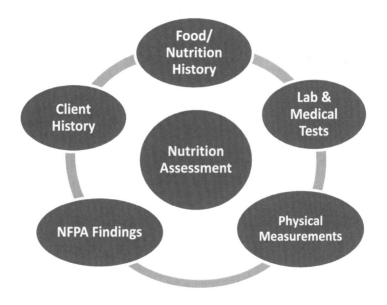

Steps to a Successful Assessment

The core of the NCP is the relationship between the client or patients and the RDN. The role of the nutrition professional is to bring science, food and technology together to address nutrition-related health problems.

There are four components of a successful assessment:

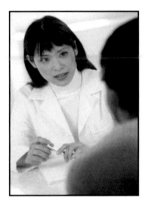

- establishing a clinician-patient relationship
- being approachable
- being an empathic listener
- allow time for self-reflection

The first step in any type of assessment is to establish a rapport with the patient. The practitioner's ability to establish a relationship with the client determines how the client or their families view the clinician. Next, the clinician must be approachable, a person the client respects and feels comfortable discussing health concerns. Practitioners must recognize that everyone has unique health concerns. As an empathic listener, the practitioner strives to see the health concerns from the patient's vantage point through verbal and nonverbal communication.

Finally, nutrition professionals should take time for self-reflection. Remember that we all have biases. The RDN's cultural and educational background may influence what he/she hears the client saying, how he/she reacts or behaves toward the patient. The RDNs personal view point may be affected by the patient's age, socioeconomic status, ethnicity or state of health.

Establishing relationships with patients is a challenge. The aim is to understand the patient's view point and nutrition-related health concerns. Then develop interventions that reflect the patient's values and health goals (Bickley, 2009).

Getting Started

If you are an experienced RDN you have a methodology for approaching each nutrition assessment. Adding NFPA to your professional toolbox will require you to adjust your thinking and preparation. In addition to the usual data gathered from the medical record, review the history and physical, nursing notes and rehabilitation therapy notes for signs and symptoms to determine which aspects of NFPA you will include as you gather data to support the nutrition-diagnosis. Note the vital signs and routine lab test results (BMP, CMP, CBC, CBG, etc). Identify your nutrition concerns from the medical record.

During the interview, you will be looking for physical signs that are consistent with the data in the medical record. For example, if the patient has a diagnosis of congestive heart failure and an elevated NT-pro-BNP, check closely for signs of edema and anasarca.

When you enter the room, introduce yourself and shake hands, if appropriate. The hand shake will give you a glimpse of the patient's strength, body temperature, presence of edema in hands, general skin condition, etc. Ask questions related to health and nutrition history and specific concerns about food, beverages and health. Once you get a sense of their food and nutrition history, explain what you would like to do. Ask the patient's permission to exam the specific areas of the body that may reflect nutrition status before starting. Watch for signs of discomfort.

Signs vs. Symptoms

Signs and symptoms are not the same thing. Signs are what the doctor or other clinician observes that can verified with objective data. Symptoms are what the patient experiences and reports to the medical team. Symptoms are subjective and reflect how the patient is experiencing the injury, illness or disease. It is important to remember that sometimes what you observe may not be consistent with the data in the medical record. Inconsistencies may be due to documentation errors or changes in condition.

Standard and Universal Precautions

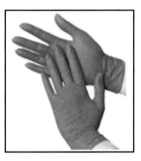

Be sure to use standard and universal precautions to protect the patient and yourself from the spread of disease. The Centers for Disease Control and Prevention (CDC) have issued several guidelines available at the CDC web sites.

Universal precautions are a set of guidelines designed to prevent transmission of bloodborne pathogens such as human immunodeficiency virus and hepatitis B virus. Standard and MRSA precautions are guidelines apply to all patients in all settings. They are designed to prevent the transmission of infectious agents via blood, body fluids, non-intact skin, secretions, excretions and mucous membranes. These guidelines include hand hygiene, when to use gloves, gowns, eye, mouth and nose protection, respiratory hygiene and cough etiquette etc. Refer to your healthcare facility's policy and procedure manual for more information. The Director of Nursing or Staff Development Coordinator may have training modules for staff to complete before hands on assessments are initiated (Bickley, 2009).

Systems Approach to Physical Assessment
There are two categories of physical assessments: comprehensive and focused. A comprehensive assessment reviews all the body systems. A focused assessment reviews selected body systems. NFPA is a focused assessment because it only addresses specific concerns or symptoms including:

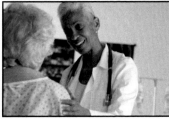

- Overall appearance
- Vital signs
- Skin
- Digestive system
- Nerves and cognition
- Cardiopulmonary system
- Extremities, muscles & bones
- HEENT (head, eyes, ears, nose, throat)

Cardinal Techniques of Physical Exam
There are four cardinal or classic techniques of a physical exam. Refer to Figures 2.3-2.9.

- **Inspection-** Close observation of the details of the patient's appearance, behavior, and movement such as facial expression, mood, body habitus, conditioning, skin color, edema, etc. In the focused observation use the senses of sight, smell, and hearing.

- **Palpation-** Tactile examination to feel pulsations and vibrations. Use the palmar fingers or fingertip pads to assess areas of skin elevation, depression, texture, size, temperature, tenderness, and mobility. For NFPA, assessing for edema, skin warmth, texture, tenderness etc.

• **Percussion-** Assessment of sounds to determine body organ borders, shape, and position. Use of the striking or plexlor finger (usually the third finger on dominant hand) to deliver a rapid tap or blow against the distal pleximeter finger (usually the third finger on non-dominant hand) laid against the surface of the chest or abdomen to evoke a sound wave from underlying tissue. The sound wave generates a tactile vibration against the pleximeter finger.

• **Auscultation-** Use of the naked ear or the bell (hollow cup) or diaphragm (flat disc) of the stethoscope to listen to body sounds (e.g., heart and lung sounds, bowel sounds, blood vessels). The bell transmits low frequency sounds while the diaphragm transmits higher frequency sounds.

Inspection and palpation are the two techniques used most often in NFPA. RDNs can be trained in using percussion and auscultation. Additional hands-on supervised clinical experience is required to learn to interpret findings (Bickley, 2009).

Collaborative Assessments

In some cases, you may need to invite another healthcare team member to assist with the assessment. For example, a patient with pressure ulcers has dressing changes periodically. Arrange for your assessment of the skin condition at the same time the nurse is doing a dressing change. If schedules are incompatible, you can use the data gathered by the wound care nurse. The more opportunities you take to assess changes in physical status, the more confident you will be in doing NFPA.

Figures 2.3-2.9. Cardinal Techniques of Physical Exam

Figures 2.3.-2.4. Inspection

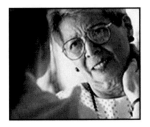 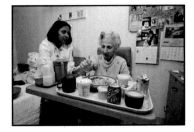

Figures 2.5.-2.6. Palpation

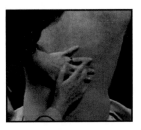 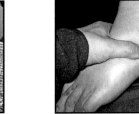

Figures 2.7.-2.8. Percussion

 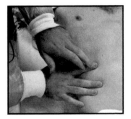

Figure 2.9. Auscultation

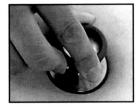

Steps in Clinical Reasoning

Clinical reasoning is the backbone of NCP. In doing physical assessments, these are the steps in clinical reasoning:

- Identify abnormal findings or symptoms
- Localize the findings anatomically
- Interpret findings in terms of probable process
- Make hypothesis about the nature of the patient's problem
- Test the hypothesis and establish a working diagnosis
- Develop a plan agreeable to the patient (Bickley, 2009)

Steps in Clinical Reasoning Using NFPA

- Identify abnormal findings or symptoms
    Examples:
    - Low hemoglobin, hematocrit, elevated MCV, diagnosis mild cognitive impairment
    - Diet history and recall indicate patient prefers vegetables and breads, dislikes milk, meat and eggs
- Localize the findings anatomically
    Example:
    - Identify physical signs of anemia, numbness in feet or hands, beefy red tongue
- Interpret findings in terms of probable process
    Example:
    - Labs, health history, diet history and physical signs that suggest nutritional anemia
- Make hypothesis about the nature of the patient's problem
    Example:
    - Nutrition diagnoses that address dietary history, labs and NFPA findings
- Test the hypothesis and establish a working diagnosis
    Example:
    - Request lab work for serum vitamin B12, folate methylmalonic acid

- Develop a plan agreeable to the patient
  Example:
  - Nutrition interventions specific to nutrition diagnosis

Clinical Nutrition Pearls: NFPA

NFPA adds a global perspective to your nutrition assessment. Nutrition diagnoses typically used in conjunction with NFPA data include excessive or suboptimal intake of sodium, excessive or suboptimal intake of other micro and macronutrients, fluid, parenteral/enteral nutrition, overweight/obesity, underweight, unintentional weight loss. Domains of intervention commonly used include food and nutrient delivery, nutrition education, nutrition counseling and coordination of care (ADA, 2011).

References

ADA. International dietetics & nutrition terminology reference manual. Chicago, IL: ADA, 2011.

ADA Practice Applications. Nutrition care process and model part I: the 2008 update. *JADA*. 2008:108:1113–1117.

Academy's Quality Management Committee. ADA revised 2008 standards of practice for registered dietitians in nutrition care; standards of professional performance for registered dietitians; standards of practice for dietetic technicians, registered, in nutrition care; and standards of professional performance for dietetic technicians, registered. *JADA*. 2008;108:1538–1542.e9.

Bickley,L. Bates Guide to physical examination, 10th ed. Philadelphia,PA: Lippincott, 2009.

Chapter 3

Overall Appearance & Vital Signs

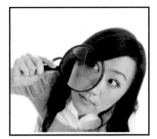

When initiating a NFPA, start with a general survey of overall appearance. The characteristics the nutrition professional is looking for are things that suggest a nutrient deficiency, nutrient toxicity or anything that negatively impacts the ability to eat food or drink fluids by mouth. Start by observing the person globally, then focus on parts of the body from head to toe (ADA, 2011).

Some questions to consider as you assess overall appearance. A more detailed discussion of these aspects of NFPA findings is included in subsequent chapters.

First Impressions
- What is the apparent state of health?
- Is the patient acutely or chronically ill?
- Is the patient frail or fit and robust?
- What is the level of consciousness?
- Is the patient awake, alert, confused, anxious?
- Does the patient show signs of physical distress?
- Does the patient have labored breathing?
- What is the person's posture?
- Do you notice any unexpected odors such as the fruity aroma of diabetes or alcohol or marijuana?
- How is the person dressed?

• Is the clothing appropriate for the season of the year and room temperature? Cold intolerance may be related to hypothyroidism or nutritional anemia.
• If the patient is wearing shoes, have the toes been cut out? Are the laces tied? Untied laces may indicate pedal edema.
• Is the patient wearing slippers? Cut out holes and slippers may indicate gout or foot ulcers. Slippers may indicate pedal edema.
• Are there any involuntary movements or signs of paralysis?
• Look at the face and hands. What does the color of the skin suggest? Pallor, jaundice, cyanosis or healthy?
• Look at the hair and fingernails for signs of nutrient deficiencies or toxicities. Changes in hair and nails can be related to medications.
• Look at the mouth, teeth and gums for signs of nutrient deficiencies.
• Listen to the patient talking. Do the dentures 'click' while the person is speaking (suggests poorly fitting dentures possible related to unplanned weight loss)?

Next, focus on specific aspects of the overall appearance. The initial survey of the patient for physical signs of nutrient deficiencies will direct the hands-on portion of the NFPA.

Body Habitus
• What is the body type or physique?
• Is the patient ectomorphic, mesomorphic or endomorphic?
• Is the BMI consistent with visual assessment of habitus?
• How does the patient describe their appetite?
• Is the self-reported appetite consistent with visual assessment of habitus?

Cushingoid Appearance
• Does the patient have an appearance that would be expected in a person with Cushing's disease (condition of pituitary gland where the body overproduces cortisol)?
• Does the patient have fatty tissue deposits, particularly around the midsection and upper back?
• Does the patient have a 'moon face'? (fatty deposits on face) Note: May be due to long-term steroid use.
• Does the patient have a 'buffalo hump'? (fatty deposits between the shoulders)
• Does the patient have thin fragile skin that bruises easily?
• Observe any slow healing cuts, insect bites or infections?

Amputations
• Does the patient have an amputation?
• Is the amputation consistent with the documentation in the medical record?
• Is the stump healed?
• If not, do you see signs of infection or smell strong odors?

Body Language
• What are the verbal/nonverbal messages related to food?
• What are the verbal/nonverbal messages related to health?
• What are the verbal/nonverbal messages related to fitness etc?
• What are the verbal/nonverbal messages related to preventive medicine/health promotion?

Affect
• Does the patient show signs of emotional distress?
• Does the patient seem depressed, inexpressive or exhibit a flat affect?
• Is the patient overly anxious?

Ability to Communicate
- Is the patient able to communicate?
- Is there a language barrier?
- Is the patient aphasic?
- Garbled language?
- Easily short of breath?
- Can the person hear you speaking?
- Does the patient answer questions appropriately?
- Does the patient project signs of readiness to make lifestyle changes?

Tanner Stage (children and teens)
- Is the developmental age consistent with chronological age?
- Are there signs of nutrient deficiencies that may have contributed to delayed growth and development?
- Are their signs of developmental delays that impact food intake?

Figure 3.1. Tanner Stage of Development

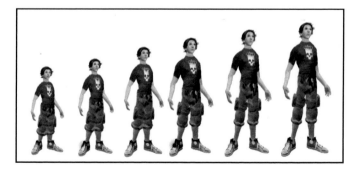

What is your first impression of these patients? What do you observe that requires more assessment and might be related to a nutrition diagnosis? Key at end of chapter.

Figure 3.2.　　　　　　　**Figure 3.3.**

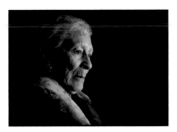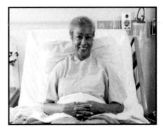

Figure 3.4.　　　　　　　**Figure 3.5.**

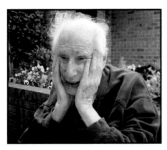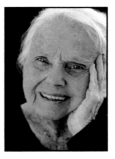

Figure 3.6.　　　　　　　**Figure 3.7.**

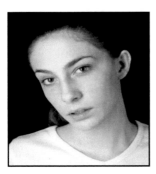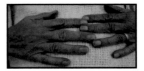

What is your first impression of these patients? What do you observe that requires more assessment and might be related to a nutrition diagnosis? Key at end of chapter.

Figure 3.8.

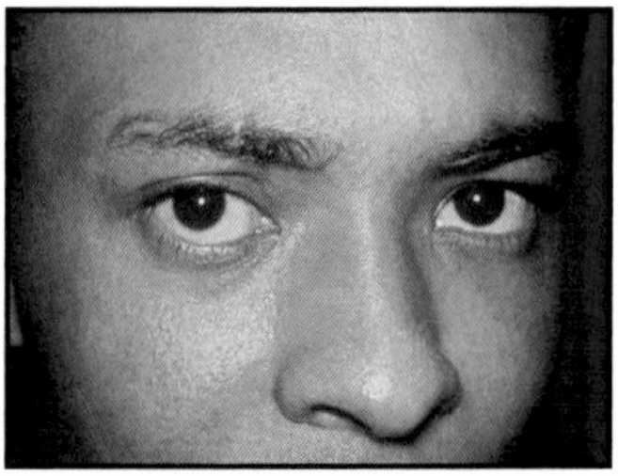

Figure 3.9.

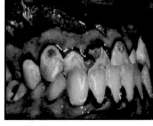

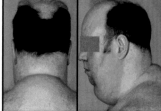

Figure 3.10.

Figure 3.11.

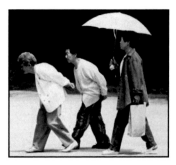

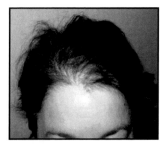

Figure 3.12.

Figure 3.13.

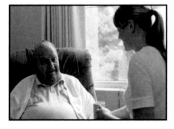

What is your first impression of these patients? What do you observe that requires more assessment and might be related to a nutrition diagnosis? Key at end of chapter.

Figure 3.14.

Figure 3.15.

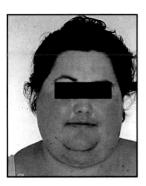

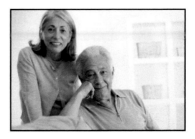

Figure 3.16.

Figure 3.17.

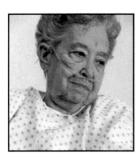

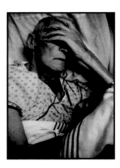

Figure 3.18.

Figure 3.19.

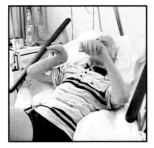

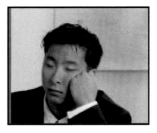

What is your first impression of these patients? What do you observe that requires more assessment and might be related to a nutrition diagnosis? Key at end of chapter.

Figure 3.20.

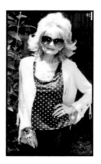

Figure 3.21.

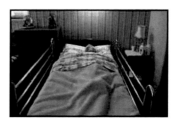

Figure 3.22.

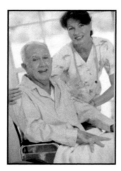

Figure 3.23.

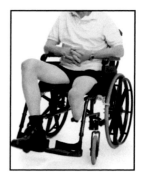

Figure 3.24.

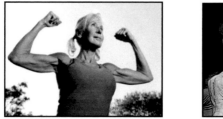

Figure 3.25.

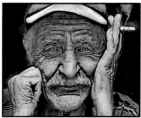

Vital Signs

Vital signs are signs of life. These are objective measures used to determine if a person is alive. Vital signs are typically assessed by nurses, medical or nursing assistants. RDNs who are trained and demonstrate competency in these assessment skills may also assess vital signs. RDNs use vital signs data recorded in the medical record to identify trends and patterns of data (Stankorb,2010; Stieber, 2011).

The purpose of recording vital signs is to establish a medical baseline upon admission to a hospital, clinic, or other encounter with a health care provider. The vital signs are compared with normal ranges for a person's age and medical condition. Based on these results, decisions are made regarding further actions to be taken.

Vital Signs include:

Figure 3.26. Blood Pressure

- Blood pressure (mm Hg)
- Heart rate (beats/min)
- Respiratory rate (breaths/min)
- Oxygen saturation (percentage)
- Temperature (degrees)

Abnormal findings may be related to injury, disease, misuse of medications, herbal or complementary products

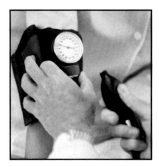

Vital Signs: Blood Pressure

Blood pressure is the force of blood against the walls of arteries. Blood pressure is recorded as two numbers—the systolic pressure (as the heart beats) over the diastolic pressure (as the heart relaxes between beats). The measurement is written one above or before the other, with the systolic number on top and the diastolic number on the bottom. The systolic number is the higher of the two numbers. Blood pressure can change from minute to minute with changes in posture, exercise, stress or sleep. It should normally be less than 120/80 mm Hg (less than 120 systolic AND less than 80 diastolic) for an adult age 20 or over.

Hypertension

A single high reading does not necessarily mean that the patient has high blood pressure or hypertension. However, if readings stay at 140/90 mm Hg or above (systolic 140 or above OR diastolic 90 or above) over time, a treatment plan including medical nutrition therapy should be considered.

Current research suggests that an elevated systolic blood pressure is a major risk factor for cardiovascular disease for individuals over 50 years old. Typically, systolic blood pressure rises steadily with age due to increasing stiffness of large arteries, long-term build-up of plaque, and increased incidence of cardiac and vascular disease (Messerli, 2009).

Seventh Report of the Joint National Committee on Prevention, Detection, Evaluation, and Treatment of High Blood Pressure (2003) recommends using the mean of two or more measured seated blood pressure readings taken on two or more days for a diagnosis of hypertension. For individuals with a diagnosis of hypertension, diabetes or renal disease the blood pressure goal is < 130/80 mm Hg. Table 3.1 notes the current blood pressure classifications for adults older than 18 years (NHLBI, 2004).

'White-coat' hypertension is defined as elevated blood pressure when the doctor checks the blood pressure, but normal the rest of the time. It is a common occurrence in about one in six adults and once thought to be medically insignificant. Other individuals have 'masked' hypertension in which blood pressure readings are normal in a medical setting, but sporadically high in real life. Both 'white-coat' and 'masked' hypertension have been associated with increased risk of developing sustained hypertension (AHA, 2009; Mancia, 2009).

Table.3.1. Blood Pressure Classifications

BP Category	Systolic mm Hg		Diastolic mm Hg
Normal	< 120	And	< 80
Pre-hypertension	120-139	Or	80-90
High blood pressure Hypertension Stage I	140-159	Or	90-99
High blood pressure Hypertension Stage II	160 or higher	Or	100 or higher
Hypertensive Crisis	>180	Or	>110

JNC7 Prevention, Detection, Evaluation, and Treatment of High Blood Pressure, 2003.

Hypotension

Low blood pressure is defined primarily by signs and symptoms of low blood flow and not by a specific blood pressure number. Some individuals routinely have blood pressures of 90/50 mm Hg with no symptoms and therefore do not have low blood pressure. However, others who normally have higher blood pressures may develop symptoms of low blood pressure if their blood pressure drops to 100/60 mm Hg.

Orthostatic hypotension is the term used to describe the fall in blood pressure when a person stands. When a person stands up, baroreceptors in the carotid arteries and aorta sense a drop in blood pressure because gravity causes blood to flow towards the legs. The sympathetic nervous system is stimulated causing the heart rate to increase and the heart to pump more blood to the brain and other organs.

Normally the systolic blood pressure drops slightly and the diastolic pressure rises slightly when a person stands up. Orthostatic hypotension is a drop in systolic blood pressure of > or= 20 mm Hg or in diastolic blood pressure of > or = to 10 mm Hg within 3 minutes of standing.

Symptoms of orthostatic hypotension include dizziness, feeling light headed or passing out. It is not a disease or a complaint from an individual. It is an abnormal change in blood pressure and heart rate associated with an illness, prolonged bed rest, dehydration, moderate to severe blood loss or a side effect of some medications (Bickley, 2009).

Pulse Pressure
Pulse pressure is the numerical difference between systolic and diastolic pressure. For example, BP 140/90 mm Hg, the pulse pressure is 50. Generally speaking a pulse pressure greater than 40-60 mm Hg is abnormal. A high pulse pressure may be a strong predictor of heart problems, especially in older adults. A pulse pressure lower than 40 mm Hg may suggest poor heart function (Bickley, 2009).

The most important cause of elevated pulse pressure is stiffness of the aorta. The stiffness may be due to hypertension or atherosclerosis. The greater the pulse pressure, the stiffer and more damaged the vessels are thought to be. Severe iron deficiency anemia and hyperthyroidism can increase pulse pressure as well.

Results of several longitudinal studies in older patients with hypertension indicate that a high pulse pressure is a sensitive marker for carotid artery stenosis, which increases the risk of stroke, coronary heart disease, and sudden death (Benetos, 2010; Roman, 2009). Treating high blood pressure usually reduces pulse pressure concurrently.

EXAMPLE 3.1.
Sam has the following blood pressure readings. What is his average pulse pressure? How would you interpret the data? 155/90 mm Hg 190/100 mm Hg 135/70 mm Hg **Answer:** 155/90   155-90= 65 190/100 190-100=90 135/70   135-70=65 65 + 90 + 65 = 190/3 = 63 His average pulse pressure is above the normal range.

Vital Signs: Heart Rate

Heart rate is determined by the number of heartbeats per unit of time, typically expressed as beats per minute (BPM). The range for normal resting heart rate is 50-100 BPM. Normal resting heart rate for athletes is 40-60 BPM As a general rule, the lower the resting heart rate, the more efficient the heart function and the better cardiovascular fitness. There are many factors that can affect heart rate including activity level, fitness level, air temperature, body position, emotions, body size and medication use.

The pulse rate can be measured at any point on the body where an artery's pulsation is transmitted to the surface when it is compressed against an underlying structure like bone. The radial pulse at the wrist is the most common site to measure heart rate. To take a pulse, press the pads of the index and middle fingers on the radial artery until maximal pulsation is detected. If the rhythm is regular, count the rate for 10 seconds and multiply by 6 or 30 seconds and multiply by 2. If the rate seems very slow or very fast, count it for 60 seconds. The thumb should not be used for measuring another person's heart rate, as its strong pulse may interfere with discriminating the site of pulsation (Bickley, 2009). See Figure 3.27.

Tachycardia is a resting heart rate of > 100 BPM. Bradycardia is a resting heart rate at < 60 BPM with other signs and symptoms such as fainting, dizziness or shortness of breath. Arrhythmia or dysrhythmia are an irregular or abnormal heart beat. Symptoms of arrhythmias may mot be detected during a physical exam. Stress or illness may trigger symptoms associated with arrhythmias including palpitations, fluttering, feeling that heart is racing, pounding in the chest, dizziness, shortness of breath, chest discomfort and weakness or fatigue.

Vital Signs: Respiratory Rate & Oxygen Saturation
Respiratory rate is the number of breaths per minute. The normal rate is about 14-20 per minute in adults. Observe respiratory rate by counting how many times the chest rises or breaths per minute. Every effort should be made to prevent the patient from becoming aware that their breathing is being checked. Respiration rates may increase with fever, illness, and with other medical conditions. Respiratory patterns are observed in terms of rate, depth and regularity. Terms commonly used to describe respiratory rate are noted in Table 3.2 (Bickley, 2009).

Oxygen saturation (SpO2) is another measure of respiratory health. It is an indicator of the percentage of hemoglobin saturated with oxygen at the time of the measurement. The reading, obtained through pulse oximetry, uses a light sensor containing two sources of light (red and infrared) that are absorbed by hemoglobin and transmitted through tissues to a photodetector.

The amount of light transmitted through the tissue is then converted to a digital value representing the percentage of hemoglobin saturated with oxygen. Normal oxygen saturation values are 97% to 99% in the healthy individual. An oxygen saturation value of 95% is clinically accepted in a patient with a normal hemoglobin level. Oxygen saturation of 90 percent or less will negatively impact wound healing. (Demling, 2003). Oxygen saturation does not indicate the patient's ability to ventilate or blow off CO_2.

Table 3.2. Descriptors of Respiratory Rate

Descriptors of Respiratory Rate	Definitions
Bradypnea	Slow breathing
Tachypnea	Rapid, shallow breathing
Hyperpnea	Rapid deep breathing
Obstructive breathing	Prolonged breathing

Figure 3.27. Heart Rate   **Figure 3.28.** Oximeter

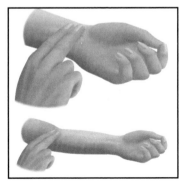
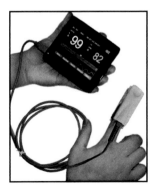

It is important to note that patients with any discoloration of the nail bed can affect the transmission of light through the digit. Dark nail polish and bruising under the nail can severely limit the transmission of light and result in an artificially decreased SpO2 value (Bickley, 2009).

Vital Signs: Temperature
The average oral body temperature is usually quoted at 98.6 degrees F, however it fluctuates considerably. Normal body temperature in healthy adults may range from 97.8 degrees Fahrenheit (F) (or 36.5 degrees Celsius) to 99 degrees F (or 37.2 degrees Celsius). Temperatures tend to be lower in the morning than in the evening. Elevated body temperature is referred to as fever or pyrexia. Causes of fever include infection, injuries, surgery and a variety of disorders. A fever is indicated when body temperature rises above 98.6° F orally or 99.8° F rectally, according to the American Medical Association. Hypothermia or low body temperature is defined as a drop in body temperature below 95° F. The chief cause of hypothermia is exposure to cold. It can also be due to paralysis, starvation, hypothyroidism and hypoglycemia or other disorders. Elderly patients are more susceptible to hypothermia than younger and middle aged adults and are less likely to develop a fever (Bickley, 2009).

Practical Applications for NFPA: Hypertension
In the U.S. and most other developed countries, blood pressure slowly rises with age. The age-related increase in blood pressure begins early in childhood and increases thereafter. According to national survey data (1999-2004), nearly a third (32%) of adult Americans have hypertension, and roughly another third are pre-hypertensive (Wang, 2004). These data also show that the prevalence of hypertension is increasing. Rates of controlled hypertension

remain low (< 40%) but are improving slightly (Cutler, 2008). Since blood pressure generally increases with age, hypertension typically occurs in middle-aged and older adults. Adults 50 years of age and older now have a 90 percent lifetime risk of becoming hypertensive (Vasan, 2002).

Some populations are disproportionately affected by hypertension and its adverse health outcomes. For example, pre-hypertensive individuals are at high risk of developing hypertension (Vasan, 2001). Individuals of African heritage generally have higher blood pressure than do other racial-ethnic groups in the U.S. (Fields, 2004). Individuals of African heritage also have a higher risk of blood pressure-related complications, particularly stroke (Ayala, 2001; Giles, 1995) and kidney failure (Klag, 1996).

Research has demonstrated that lowering sodium intake and increasing potassium intake reduces blood pressure and its consequences of heart disease and stroke. However, not everyone benefits equally from reducing sodium and increasing potassium intake. Individuals who experience the greatest benefit from lowering sodium intake have been classified as 'salt or sodium sensitive.' Typically these are individuals with hypertension, diabetes, and chronic kidney disease. They tend to be middle-aged and older adults. Individuals of African heritage tend to be more sensitive to sodium than Caucasian adults. Genetic factors also influence the blood pressure response to sodium. Each of the 14 identified genes that affect blood pressure affects renal sodium handling. Such evidence provides indirect support of an etiologic role of sodium in blood pressure homeostasis (Lifton, 2002; IOM, 2010).

The 2010 *Dietary Guidelines for Americans (DGA)* includes a recommendation to address the evidence-based diet-blood pressure relationship (USDA, 2010).

Reduce daily sodium intake to less than 2,300 milligrams (mg) and further reduce intake to 1,500 mg among persons who are 51 and older and those of any age who are African American or have hypertension, diabetes, or chronic kidney disease. The 1,500 mg recommendation applies to about half of the U.S. population, including children, and the majority of adults

The 2010 *DGA* did not include specific recommendations for potassium intake since the evidence linking higher intakes to lower blood pressure was inconsistent. The Institute of Medicine (IOM, 2005) set the AI (adequate intakes) for potassium for adults at 4700 mg/day and no UL (upper tolerable limit) was set. Individuals with impaired potassium excretion should be evaluated by the RDN.

Nutrition professionals using NFPA may determine that elevated blood pressure findings, diagnosis of hypertension, diabetes or chronic kidney disease, presence of edema support nutrition diagnosis specific to sodium and potassium intake. Other possible nutrition diagnoses include excessive bioactive substance intake or excessive alcohol intake. Changes in blood pressure, reduced edema and dietary compliance provide insightful information for monitoring and evaluating outcomes.

Practical Applications for NFPA: Hypotension
Hypotension is less often observed in medical settings. When blood pressure is lower than normal it may be due to dehydration. Nutrition professionals using NFPA may determine that lower than normal blood pressure readings along with other risk factors associated with dehydration

support nutrition diagnoses related to insufficient water intake.

Practical Applications for NFPA: Heart Rate

Abnormal heart rate due tachycardia, bradycardia, or arrhythmias can negatively impact the ability to eat. Signs and symptoms of abnormalities include feeling light headed, fainting, dizziness, shortness of breath, chest discomfort, fatigue, and weakness. Nutrition professionals using NFPA may determine that data documenting abnormal heart rate support nutrition diagnoses related to involuntary weight loss, inadequate intakes and interventions related to food and nutrient delivery at meals, feeding assistance, use of medical food supplements and other interventions as deemed appropriate.

Target heart rate is a measure of an individual's level of fitness. Nutrition professionals using exercise as a NCP intervention may find it helpful to track target heart rate zone as a measure of compliance and improved physical fitness. Desirable Target Heart Rate Zones are based on age. The maximum heart rate for men is about 220 minus chronological age. The maximum heart rate for women is about 226 minus chronological age (Bickley, 2009).

Practical Applications for NFPA: Respiratory Rate & Oxygen Saturation

Individuals with cardiovascular and pulmonary disorders often experience shortness of breath, have abnormal breathing patterns, and may require supplemental oxygen. The process of eating, chewing the food and talking during a meal may result in increased energy expenditure, fatigue and dyspnea. Individuals may report 'I can't catch my breath' or 'I'm too tired to eat a full meal.' Others may fall asleep at meal time. Signs and symptoms of respiratory illness may be due to aspiration pneumonia. Collaborative assessments with the speech pathologist may reveal dysphagia.

Oxygen saturation of 95 percent or greater is essential for wound healing. Individuals with poor wound healing who have oxygen saturation levels less than 90 percent may benefit from supplemental oxygen (Demling, 2003).

Nutrition professionals using NFPA may determine that abnormal respiratory findings support nutrition diagnosis specific to suboptimal nutrient intake, biting/chewing difficulty, unintended weight loss.

Practical Applications for NFPA: Temperature
Abnormal body temperatures suggest a change in health status which may in turn result in decreased appetite. In elderly patients, a decreased appetite may be a better indicator of a change in health status than body temperature since elders are less likely to spike a fever.

Clinical Nutrition Pearls: Appearance & Vital Signs
Everyone observes different things doing NFPA. The purposes of gathering NFPA data are to support nutrition diagnoses and to serve as a benchmark for monitoring and evaluation. Nutrition diagnoses often used in conjunction with vital signs include excessive or suboptimal intake of sodium and other vitamins and minerals, excessive bioactive substance intake, excessive alcohol intake, underweight, unintentional weight loss, or gain, overweight or obesity.

Always corroborate your observations and findings with other members of the healthcare team. Look for patterns in the vital sign data you are collecting. The timing of meals or the nutrient composition of meals may be impacting the data and signal changes in the Nutrition Prescription.

Key to exercise on pages 25-28. Listed below are some possible observations from Figures 3.2-3.25.

3.2.- flat affect, elderly, undernourished

3.3. - healthy, robust, alert, awake, older adult

3.4. - confused, unkept, undernourished, frail, ectomorphic body type

3.5. – elderly, healthy, alert, awake

3.6. – young adult, pallor, possible nutritional anemia

3.7. - bluish nails, possible cyanosis

3.8. - yellowish sclera, possible jaundice

3.9. - endomorphic body type, Cushingoid appearance, buffalo hump, possible metabolic syndrome

3.10. - unhealthy gums and teeth

3.11. - hair loss

3.12. - stages of bone loss from healthy bone status on far right female, osteopenia or osteoporosis on middle and far left female

3.13. - endomorphic body type, apple shaped body

3.14 - endomorphic body type, Cushingoid appearance, possible metabolic syndrome

3.15. - mesomorphic older couple, robust, healthy, well nourished

3.16. - elder, requires oxygen, may have fatigue issues during eating, appears depressed

3.17. - elder, fatigue, undernourished, depressed, anxious, frail

3.18. - male, adult, contractures that may impact ability to eat independently

3.19. – young adult, fatigued, pallor, possible nutritional anemia

3.20. – ectomorphic body type, older adult, pallor, frail, undernourished

3.21. – ectomorphic body type, elderly, possible cold intolerance

3.22. – mesomorphic body type, well-nourished, alert, elder

3.23. - below the knee amputation

3.24. - robust, fit adult, mesomorphic body type

3.25. - smoker, thin face, undernourished, may have health issues related to smoking

References

ADA. *International dietetics & nutrition terminology reference manual.* Chicago, IL: ADA, 2011.

American Heart Association. White-coat, masked hypertension raises risk of sustained high blood pressure [press release]. June 29, 2009.

Ayala C, Greenlund KJ, Croft JB, Keenan NL. Racial/ethnic disparities in mortality by stroke subtype in the United States, 1995-1998. *Am J Epidemiol.* 2001 Dec 1;154(11):1057-63.

Benetos A, et al. Pulse pressure amplification: A mechanical biomarker of cardiovascular disease risk. *Journal of the American College of Cardiology.* 2010;55:1032.

Bickley,L. *Bates guide to physical examination*, 10th ed. Philadelphia,PA: Lippincott, 2009.

Cutler JA, Sorlie P. Trends in hypertension prevalence, awareness, treatment, and control rates in United States adults between 1988-1994 and 1999-2004. *Hypertension.* 2008 Nov;52(5):818-27.

Demling, R.H., DeSanti, L, (2003). Involuntary weight loss and the non-healing cutaneous wound. Medscape Clinical Update. Accessed June 2009. http://www.mwdscape.com/viewprogram/714_pnt.

Fields LE, Burt VL. The burden of adult hypertension in the United States 1999 to 2000: a rising tide. *Hypertension.* 2004 Oct;44(4):398-404.

Giles WH, Kittner SJ, Hebel J. Determinants of black-white differences in the risk of cerebral infarction. The National Health and Nutrition Examination Survey Epidemiologic Follow-up Study. *Arch Intern Med.* 1995 Jun 26;155(12):1319-24.

Institute of Medicine. *Dietary Reference Intakes for Water, Potassium, Sodium, Chloride, and Sulfate.* Washington, DC: The National Academies Press; 2005.

Institute of Medicine. *Strategies to Reduce Sodium Intake in the United States.* Washington, DC. The National Academies Press; 2010.

Klag MJ, Whelton PK, Randall B. Blood pressure and end-stage renal disease in men. *N Engl J Med.* 1996 Jan 4;334(1):13-8.

Lifton RP, Wilson FH. Salt and blood pressure: new insight from human genetic studies. *Cold Spring Harb Symp Quant Biol.* 2002;67:445-50.

Mancia G, Bombelli M, Facchetti R, et al. Long-term risk of sustained hypertension in white-coat or masked hypertension. *Hypertension* 2009; 54:00-00 DOI: 10.1161/HYPERTENSIO-Naha.109.129882. Available at: http://hyper.ahajournals.org/.

Messerli F, Makani H. Relentless progression towards sustained hypertension. *Hypertension* 2009; DOI: 10.1161/HYPERTENSIO-Naha.109.132936. Available at: http://hyper.ahajournals.org/.

National Heart, Lung, and Blood Institute (NHLBI). The seventh report of the Joint National Committee on prevention, detection, evaluation, and the treatment of high blood pressure. NIH Publication No. 04-5230. Bethesda, MD: National Heart Lung, Blood Institute. 2004.

Roman MJ, et al. High central pulse pressure is independently associated with adverse cardiovascular outcome. *Journal of the American College of Cardiology.* 2009;54:1730.

Stankorb SM, Rigassio-Radler D, Khan H, Touger-Decker R. Nutrition-focused physical examination practices of registered dietitians. *Top Clin Nutr.* 2010;25:335–344.

Stieber,M Scope of practice and legal issues in nutrition-focused physical examination. *Support Line* April, 2011, 2-6.

The Seventh Report of the Joint National Committee on Prevention, Detection, Evaluation, and Treatment of High Blood Pressure. *JAMA* 2003;289:2560–71.

U.S. Department of Agriculture and U.S. Department of Health and Human Services. Dietary Guidelines for Americans, 2010. 7th Edition, Washington, DC: U.S. Government Printing Office, December 2010. http://health.gov/dietaryguidelines/dga2010/ DietaryGuidelines2010.pdf

Vasan RS, Beiser A, Seshadri S, Larson MG, Kannel WB, D'Agostino RB, Levy D. Residual lifetime risk for developing hypertension in middle-aged women and men: The Framingham Heart Study. *JAMA*. 2002 Feb 27;287(8):1003-10.

Vasan RS, Larson MG, Leip EP, Evans JC, O'Donnell CJ, Kannel WB, Levy D. Impact of high-normal blood pressure on the risk of cardiovascular disease. *N Engl J Med*. 2001 Nov 1;345(18):1291-7.

Wang Y, Wang QJ. The prevalence of prehypertension and hypertension among U.S. adults according to the new joint national committee guidelines: New challenges of the old problem. *Arch Intern Med*. 2004; 164:2126–2134.

Chapter 4
Tools for Assessing Malnutrition

Assessment for malnutrition begins with using validated screening tools. For those identified at risk for malnutrition, use the new recommendations from the Academy's Malnutrition Workgroup and ASPEN Malnutrition Task Force. The objective of the collaborative work of the Academy's & ASPEN was to standardized definitions, coding, and to define multiple characteristics used to diagnose malnutrition. In addition, the consensus groups examined the emerging role of inflammation and its influence on assessment parameters, response to nutrition intervention, and identification of anti-inflammatory interventions/nutrition interventions. The characteristics of malnutrition include descriptors for severe and non-severe malnutrition. Note that non-severe does NOT mean not urgent. Non-severe means moderate malnutrition.

Screening for Malnutrition
Nutrition screening should be done on every admission. However, not every patient with a positive screen will meet the criteria for malnutrition. Lengthy surgeries, complex medical conditions, diagnostic testing and complications increase the risk of developing malnutrition during a hospitalization or extended care stay.

Use valid screening tools to identify malnutrition such as the Full Mini Nutritional Assessment Tool (MNA), Mini Nutritional Assessment Tool (i.e. Short Form) (MNA) (Bauer, 2008; Kaiser, 2009, 2010), Malnutrition Screening Tool (MST), Subjective Global Assessment (SGA) Tool

(Cooper, 2002; Norman, 2005). For MST and MNA tools the answers receive weighted score. The total score triggers appropriate action. The SGA does not use a numerical scoring system. The practitioner uses clinical judgement to classify the nutrition status. The MNA screens out well-nourished older adults, but does not differentiate between the nutritionally at risk and the malnourished as the Full MNA. Each tool is described in Table 4.1.

Table 4.1. Nutrition Screening Tools

Tool	Description	Source
MST	2 question screening tool examining for weight loss and changes in appetite.	Ferguson M et al. Nutrition 1999;15, (6): 458-464. Abbott Labs
Full MNA	18 question assessment tool examining appetite, anthropometric measurements, mobility, psychosocial issues, medications, skin ulcers, food and nutrition history and self-view of health and nutrition status of elderly	Nestle Nutrition Institute www.mna-elderly.com
MNA	Short form includes 6 question assessment tool examining food intake, appetite, weight loss, mobility, acute illness or stress, dementia or depression and BMI of elderly. Calf circumference can be used instead of BMI if measures are unavailable.	Nestle Nutrition Institute www. mna-elderly.com
SGA	2 part tool examining medical history and physical exam. Medical history includes changes in weight, diet, GI symptoms, and functional capacity. Physical exam includes loss of subcutaneous fat, muscle wasting, and edema. Optional water test to evaluate for dysphagia.	Covinsky KE, et al. J Am Geriatr Soc 1999; 47:532-538.

Practical Applications for NFPA:
Characteristics of Malnutrition

The Characteristics of Malnutrition is a 'work in progress.' The characteristics are derived from an etiology based malnutrition model (Jensen, 2009, 2010; Soeters, 2009). First nutritional risk is identified based on compromised dietary intake or loss of body mass. Next, the role of inflammation is considered. If inflammation is not present, the etiology of the malnutrition is starvation related or anorexia nervosa.

Malnutrition is in the context of acute illness or injury, chronic illness or social or environmental circumstances. Acute illness or injury related malnutrition has a marked inflammatory response and is often severe. Examples of malnutrition in the context of acute illness or injury include major infection, burns, trauma, or closed head injury. Examples of malnutrition in the context of chronic illness related include organ failure, cancer, rheumatoid arthritis or sarcopenic obesity. Examples of malnutrition in the context of social or environmental circumstances include knowledge, beliefs or attitudes that negatively impact intake, factors affecting access to food or nutrition-related activities of daily living.

The characteristics of malnutrition are grouped as non-severe and severe. Table 4.2. includes the characteristics used to identify non-severe malnutrition and Table 4.3. includes the characteristics used to identify severe malnutrition (ADA, 2011). Individuals must have 2 or more characteristics for a diagnosis of malnutrition. It is expected that the characteristics used to identify malnutrition will change over time as evidence of validity accrues. The criteria are discussed in the subsequent sections.

Table 4.2. Characteristics of Non-Severe Malnutrition by Etiology (ADA, 2011)

Criteria for Non-Severe	Acute Illness or Injury	Chronic Illness or Disease	Environmental or Social Circumstances
Evidence of reduced dietary intake	>7 d intake < 75%) Total Estimated Energy Requirement	≥1 mo intake <75% Total Estimated Energy Requirement	≥3 mo intake <75% Total Estimated Energy Requirement
Unintended Weight Loss	1- 2 % in 1 wk 5 % in 1 mo 7.5 % in 3 mo	5 % in 1 mo 7.5 % in 3 mo 10 % in 6 mo 20 % in 1 yr	>5 % in 1 mo >7.5 % in 3 mo >10 % in 6 mo >20 % in 1 yr
Changes in Body Composition: Loss of Subcutaneous Fat	Mild loss	Mild loss	Mild loss
Changes in Body Composition: Muscle Loss	Mild loss	Mild loss	Mild loss
Changes in Body Composition: Fluid Accumulation	Mild edema	Mild edema	Mild edema
Reduced Grip Strength	Not applicable	Not applicable	Not applicable

Abbreviations Key:
d- days, wk- week, mo- month or months, yr- year

Table 4.3. Characteristics of Severe Malnutrition by Etiology (ADA, 2011)

Criteria for Severe	Acute Illness or Injury	Chronic Illness or Disease	Environmental or Social Circumstances
Evidence of reduced dietary intake	≥5 d intake ≤50% Total Estimated Energy Requirement	≥1 mo intake ≤75% Total Estimated Energy Requirement	≥1 mo intake ≤50% Total Estimated Energy Requirement
Unintended Weight Loss	>2 % in 1 wk >5 % in 1 mo >7.5 % in 3 mo	>5 % in 1 mo >7.5 % in 3 mo >10 % in 6 mo >20 % in 1 yr	>5 % in 1 mo >7.5 % in 3 mo >10 % in 6 mo >20 % in 1 yr
Changes in Body Composition: Loss of Subcutaneous Fat	Moderate loss	Severe loss	Severe loss
Changes in Body Composition: Muscle Loss	Moderate loss	Severe loss	Severe loss
Changes in Body Composition: Fluid Accumulation	Moderate to severe edema	Severe edema	Severe edema
Reduced Grip Strength	Measurably reduced	Measurably reduced	Measurably reduced

Abbreviations Key:
d- days, wk- week, mo- month or months, yr- year

Evidence of Reduced Dietary Intake

Evidence of reduced dietary intake is not the same as percent of food served. This characteristic refers to intake as a percent of energy requirements as determined by the

RDN. Malnutrition is the result of insufficient nutrient intake or assimilation compared to total estimated energy and nutrient requirements. The characteristic of malnutrition for energy intake compares actual food consumption as a percentage of estimated energy requirement. The characteristic of malnutrition for interpretation of weight loss includes evaluation of other clinical findings (i.e. hydration) that impact weight. Weight change assessment is reported as a percentage of weight lost from baseline or usual weight.

Malnutrition usually causes changes in body composition. RDNs can use NFPA to determine and document loss of subcutaneous fat, muscle mass or fluid accumulation. In addition, functional performance is impaired. The current characteristics of malnutrition only include reduced grip strength as an evidenced-base measurement (Bohannon, 2010; Kaburagi, 2011; Kaur, 2010). However other functional performance tests are included in subsequent sections. Work collaboratively with physical and occupational therapists to collect data on these performance tests if applicable to your patient. Contribute to the body of knowledge by doing research to examine the relationship between functional performance and nutrition status.

Characteristics of malnutrition do not include lab test results for albumin, prealbumin or C-reactive protein. These laboratory tests are measures of inflammation and are not useful in diagnosing malnutrition (Keys, 1948; Jenson, 2009; Soeters, 2009). Refer to Academy's Evidence Analysis Library under albumin/prealbumin for a summary of the evidence. http://www.adaevidencelibrary.com

It is important to differentiate between sub-optimal intakes due to iatrogenic malnutrition vs. undernourished. Many "apparently healthy" patients without prior history of malnutrition or chronic disease experience sub-optimal dietary intake and unintended weight change with acute illness or trauma. Clinical judgement is required to determine if the changes represent iatrogenic malnutrition or a previously unidentified sub-optimal nutrition status that is either non-severe or severe malnutrition.

Also note that the comparative standard for reduced dietary intake is total estimated energy requirement rather than total energy served. Most food intake records are based on percentage of foods eaten.

EXAMPLE 4.1
Ms. R, 70 year old female, 60 in., 85 lbs, BMI 17, usual wt 90 lbs. She is recovering from surgery. Nursing reports that over the last 7 days she has eaten about 50% of her meals. Nutrition Rx.: Regular Diet. Nutrient analysis of the Regular Diet indicates that average daily energy is 2000 calories. Does her intake meet the criteria for 'reduced dietary intake?' **Answer:** Refer to end of chapter.

Unintended Weight Loss

Changes in weight may be due to amputation, loss of lean body mass, loss of fluid, loss of fat, removal of a cast or other appliance that contributes to body weight. Scales provide a measure of weight changes, but the numbers are only one piece of important data. Scales need to be calibrated regularly and maintained according to the manufacturer's use and care manual. Weights taken on different scales or at different locations may document weight changes that are not clinically significant. For example weights taken at home on bathroom scales may be different from weights taken at a doctor's office.

Individuals hospitalized for planned diuresis experience significant weight loss from fluid loss. The changes in weight are intentional, desired as part of the medical management of the patient and not an indicator of malnutrition.

CMS regulated extended care facilities required to complete the MDS 3.0, are allowed to use self-reported weights, weights from a physician's office or hospital record as a benchmark to determine percentage of weight loss for a new admission Data is recorded in MDS 3.0, Section K03000 (CMS, 2011). Since self-reported weights may be inaccurate, this benchmark may need to be corroborated promptly.

EXAMPLE 4.2
Ms. R, had a CVA following her surgery and has been moved to a nursing home after 8 days in the hospital. Data at discharge from hospital: 70 yr., F, 60 in., 85 lbs, Data at the nursing home for initial MDS: 60 in., 80 lbs, usual wt 90 lbs. Does her weight change meet the requirements for 'unintended weight loss?' **Answer:** Refer to end of chapter.

Changes in Body Composition

Changes in body composition require physical assessment. The NFPA will focus on assessing for loss of subcutaneous fat, muscle wasting and fluid accumulation.

Changes in Body Composition: Loss of Subcutaneous Fat

Subcutaneous fat is the adipose tissue lying between the skin and abdominal wall. It serves as a shock absorber to the skin, is a source of stored energy and contains blood vessels and nerves. Assess for loss of subcutaneous fat overlying the ribs, orbital and triceps. Orbital fat is a semifluid adipose cushion that lines the bony orbit supporting the eye. To assess for orbital fat loss, inspect for loss of fat under the eye. The fat pad under the eye is slightly bulged in the well-nourished individual. In overweight and obese individuals, the fat pads can be large and bulging. Loss of orbital fat gives the appearance of a 'hollow eye.' In non-severe malnutrition the fat loss will be mild, with a somewhat hollow appearance and often dark circles under the eyes. In severe malnutrition, the orbital area has more pronounced fat loss giving a hollow or depressed appearance. Skin may be loose and dark circles may be evident. Also look for facial and buccal fat loss. Refer to Figures 4.1.-4.5.

Use palpation to assess for loss of fat overlying the ribs. Well-nourished individuals have some fat overlying the ribs that can be pinched between the thumb and index finger. In non-severe malnutrition the fat loss will be mild with some fat is present to pinch between the thumb and index finger. In severe malnutrition, the fat overlying the ribs has more pronounced fat loss. Rib cage and other bony structures are visually prominent under the skin. Refer to Figures 4.6.-4.8.

The triceps area of the arm is the location most identified with fat loss. Use palpation to assess for loss of fat overlying the triceps. Well-nourished individuals have some fat overlying the triceps that can be pinched between the thumb and index fingers. In non-severe malnutrition the fat loss is mild, and some fat is present to pinch between the thumb and index finger. In severe malnutrition, the fat loss is moderate to severe and the there is little to no fat overlying the triceps. Refer to Figures 4.9.-4.10.

The chest and ribs area is another site to observe for loss of fullness or loose skin. In well-nourished individuals there is ample adipose tissue covering the chest wall and ribs are not prominent. In non-severe malnutrition there is moderate fat loss, the skin may be loose and the ribs may be somewhat apparent. In severe malnutrition, the skin may appear stretched over the skeleton and ribs are prominent and well-defined.

Changes in Body Composition: Loss of Muscle
Muscle atrophy or wasting may be from inactivity, diseases of peripheral nervous system, diseases of the muscles, disease related cachexia and sarcopenia. Concurrent malnutrition exacerbates muscle atrophy. NFPA of muscle loss includes muscle volume, tone and function.

Muscle wasting can be bilateral (both sides of the body are affected) or unilateral (only one side of the body is affected). Wasting is determined by inspection and palpation for muscle volume and tone. Observe the patient straight on with arms at each side. Do the muscles look flat, concave or hollow, suggesting atrophy? Are underlying skeletal structures prominent?

Muscle tone or the residual muscle tension is the continuous and passive partial contraction of muscles. Descriptors of reduced muscle tone include flaccidity and hypotonus. Flaccidity means lack of tone or active movement. The muscles feel soft and offer no resistance to passive movement. Hypotonus refers to decreased muscle tone and is associated with increased muscle weakness.

Temporalis Muscle Wasting
The temporalis muscle attaches to the temporal bone on the side of the head above the ear. It looks similar to a scallop shell with the tendon representing the hinge of the shell. It is one of the muscles of mastication. In NFPA, look for temporal wasting or a thinning of the muscle tissue over the

temporal bones resulting in a scooping or hollowing appearance. The brow bone is prominent. In well-nourished individuals there is ample well-defined muscle. In non-severe malnutrition there is a slight depression of the temporalis muscle. In severe malnutrition, hollowing and scooping depression is apparent. Refer to Figures 4.11.-4.12.

Interosseous Muscle Wasting

Wasting of the hand can be part of generalized wasting common seen in malnutrition or it can be localized. Localized wasting may be due to nerve damage, insufficient blood supply, disuse or distal myopathy.

The palmar and dorsal interosseous muscles of the hand are found near the metacarpal bones that help to control the fingers. The dorsal interosseous muscles are between the bones of the finger. These muscles may atrophy with aging, malnutrition, rheumatoid arthritis, poliomyelitis, leprosy and amyotrophic lateral sclerosis (if it begins in the hands). Loss of hand strength can also impair all activities of daily living including meal preparation and self-feeding. Using NFPA, observe and palpate the hands for signs of dorsal interosseous muscle wasting. Note any signs of discomfort. Refer to Figures 4.13-4.14.

Upper Body Wasting: Deltoid, Pectoris and Clavicle

The upper body is more susceptible to muscle loss than other parts of the body. Loss of upper body muscle volume is independent of function. Observe the volume of pectoral, biceps and deltoid muscles. Protrusion of bone usually indicates muscle wasting. In well-nourished men the clavicle bone is not prominent, but is often visible in women. In non-severe malnutrition there is a slight protrusion of the clavicle. In severe malnutrition, the clavicle bone is prominent and protruding. Refer to Figures 4.15.-4.21.

Upper Body Wasting: Shoulder

Observe the patient straight on with arms at each side. Look for loss of roundness at the junction of the shoulder and neck and at the junction of the shoulder and arm. In well-nourished individuals the curves are rounded at the junction of the shoulder and neck and at the junction of the shoulder and arm. The acromion process (highest point of the shoulder) is not evident. In non-severe malnutrition there is a slight protrusion of the acromion process. In severe malnutrition, the acromion process is prominent or protruding suggesting significant loss of the deltoid muscle. Refer to Figures 4.22-4.23.

Upper Body Wasting: Scapula, Trapezius & Latissimus Dorsi

Observe the patient's back for signs of muscle wasting. Muscles to observe include trapezius and latissimus dorsi. The trapezius extends longitudinally from the occipital bone to the lower thoracic vertebrae and laterally to the spine of the scapula. The latissimus dorsi is the larger, flat, dorso-lateral muscle on the trunk, posterior to the arm, and partly covered by the trapezius on its median dorsal region. Refer to figures 4.18.-4.25. In well-nourished individuals the curves of the back are rounded and the shoulder blade does not protrude. In non-severe malnutrition there may be a slight protrusion of the scapula. In severe malnutrition, muscle loss is moderate to severe. The scapula is prominent or protruding suggesting significant loss of the trapezius and latissimus dorsi muscles.

Lower Body Wasting: Quadriceps & Gastrocnemius

The quadriceps femoris is a large muscle group including

the four muscles in the front of the thigh. The calf muscle that has a bulging shape is the gastrocnemius. It runs from the just above the knee to the heel. The quadriceps femoris and gastrocnemius muscles are involved in standing, walking, running and jumping. Muscle loss from inactivity or bedrest is most prominent in the lower body. Refer to Figures 4.26-4.31.

In well-nourished individuals the curves of the quadriceps femoris and gastrocnemius are full and well-defined. In non-severe malnutrition there is a mild loss of muscle. In severe malnutrition, there is moderate to severe loss of the quadriceps femoris and gastrocnemius muscles.

Changes in Body Composition: Fluid Accumulation

Fluid accumulation in body tissues or edema may be localized or generalized. All types of edema may mask weight loss and might reflect weight gain. Edema is assessed using inspection and palpation.

Edema is categorized as either pitting or non-pitting edema. Pitting edema can be identified by applying pressure to a swollen area by depressing fingertip pads to skin. If an indentation persists upon release, it is pitting edema. Common types of pitting edema are noted on Table 4.4.

Table 4.4. Types of Pitting Edema

Type of Edema	Site of Edema
Peripheral edema	legs and feet
Pedal edema	feet
Pulmonary edema	alveoli in the lungs
Ascites	abdomen
Pleural edema	lung or pleural cavity
Vulvar/Scrotal edema	gender specific pubic areas
Anasarca	overall body edema

Non-pitting edema usually affects the arms and legs. When pressure is applied to the area of fluid accumulation, an indentation does not persist. Non-pitting edema can occur in certain disorders of the lymphatic system including lymphedema after mastectomy or lymph node surgery. The two common methods for describing and assessing edema are noted in Table 4.5. Refer to Figures 4.32-4.38.

Table 4. 5. Assessment of Edema

Category	Description		Description
1+	Mild pitting, slight indentation, no perceptible swelling (2 mm)	OR	If pitting lasts 0 to 15 seconds
2+	Moderate pitting, indentation subsides rapidly (4 mm)	OR	If pitting lasts 16 to 30 seconds
3+	Deep pitting, indentation remains a short time, extremity looks swollen (6 mm)	OR	If pitting lasts 31 to 60 seconds
4+	Very deep pitting, indentation lasts a long time, extremity is very swollen (8 mm)	OR	If pitting lasts more than 60 seconds

Documenting Changes in Body Composition

During NFPA, note the frequency of each characteristic of malnutrition noted in Table 4.6 and sum the total number of changes. In well-nourished individuals, there are no evident changes in body composition. In non-severe malnutrition, 1-2 changes will be noted. In severe malnutrition, 3 or more changes will be noted.

Table 4.6. Documenting Changes in Body Composition

Frequency	Type of change
Number identified	Loss of subcutaneous fat (triceps, ribs, orbital)
Number identified	Muscle wasting (temporal, hand, upper and lower body)
Number identified	Extremity edema (hand, arm, ankle, leg)
Number identified	Vulvar/scrotal edema
Number identified	Generalized edema

EXAMPLE 4.3
Using NFPA, the RDN notes that Mrs. R has muscle wasting at the clavicle and deltoids. Her face is very thin and it appears that she has temporal muscle wasting. She does not have any fluid accumulation. Do these findings meet the criteria for 'change in body composition?' **Answer:** Refer to end of chapter.

Measures of Physical Function & Performance: Hand Grip Strength

The only measure of physical function and performance included in the current characteristics of malnutrition is for hand grip strength. Hand grip strength is determined using a dynamometer. The purpose of this test is to measure the maximum isometric strength of the hand and forearm muscles. The procedure for measuring hand grip strength and the criteria for interpreting the data is specific to each manufacturer. Generally speaking, the patient holds the dynamometer in the hand to be tested, with the arm at right angles and the elbow by the side of the body. Be sure to place the strap around the patient's wrist for safety.

Allow the patient to comfortably arrange the instrument in his/her hand. The base should rest on the heel of palm and the handle should rest on middle of four fingers.

When ready, the patient squeezes the dynamometer with maximum isometric effort holding the grip for about 5 seconds. Document the maximum reading from 3 attempts. Be sure to allow 60 seconds between measurements. Take measurements on the dominant and non-dominant hand. Use the manufacturer's standards differentiating between excellent, good, average, fair and poor performance. Presently, the strongest correlation with muscle mass and nutrition status is hand grip strength (Bohannon, 2010; Ha, 2010, Kaburagi, 2011, Norman, 2011, Pieterese, 2002; Wang, 2005). Refer to Figures 4.39-4.40.

Clinical Nutrition Pearls: Malnutrition
The current recommendation from the Academy/ ASPEN Task Forces is that the presence of two or more characteristics is required for a nutrition diagnosis of malnutrition. Nutrition professionals have further criteria to differentiate between non-severe and severe malnutrition for each characteristic. The characteristics used to identify malnutrition are a 'work in progress' and will change over time as evidence of validity accrues.

Characteristics of malnutrition include some new tools to assess nutrition status. Consult other members of medical team for guidance in refining your clinical skills to assess for different degrees of fluid accumulation and measures of hand grip strength. There are numerous tests of functional performance, but only hand grip strength has evidence based research correlating the findings to changes in nutrition status. Measuring functional performance using hand grip strength may be new skill to add to your NFPA toolbox. RDs may be able to work collaboratively with rehabilitation therapy professionals currently using hand grip strength to measure improvements in performance. In addition, rehabilitation therapists may be helpful in identifying sources of professional grade hand grips and training resources.

Malnutrition is a nutrition diagnosis. PES statements may incorporate NFPA observations specific to weight loss, changes in body composition, physical function and performance test scores and dietary data. he nutrition professional develops intervention strategies and monitoring criteria to evaluate outcomes.

Other Measures of Diminished Strength: Lower Extremity Physical Function & Performance

Evidence based measures of lower extremity physical function or performance include walking tests, stair climbing, chair rising, and balance. A score is determined for each test and summed for interpretation (Humphreys, 2002; Ha, 2010; Guralnik, 1994, 1995). These functional tests are not part of the Academy/ASPEN Characteristics of Malnutrition. However, there is evidence based research that these tests measure changes in functional status. RDNs have the opportunity to develop research projects to determine if these measures correlate with changes in nutrition status. Work collaboratively with physical therapy or occupational therapy for a better understanding of functional measures of performance.

Walk Test

The walking test requires a flat surface for walking a predetermined distance and a stopwatch. The purpose of this test is to determine the usual pace of walking and to determine a gait ordinal score. The slower a person walks, the greater the risk for mortality, nursing home admission and disability (Guralnik, 1994, 1995). Individuals who use canes or other walking aids outside of the home should be encouraged to use these aids for the walking test.

One commonly used walk test is the 8 foot or 2.44 meter test. Measure and mark a distance of 16 feet or 4.88 meters. Mark off the first 4 feet or 1.22 meters and last 4 feet or 1.22 meters. Although you ask the patient to walk the entire 16 feet or 4.88 meters, only the middle 8 feet or 2.44 meters are recorded.

The first and last 4 feet or 1.22 meters are used to eliminate periods of acceleration and deceleration. Instruct the patient to walk to a specific landmark (i.e. yellow line or other marker) as fast as he/she feels comfortable and safe.

Timing starts when the first part of either lower extremity passes the 4 foot mark or 1.22 meter mark. Timing ends when the first part of either lower extremity passes the 12 foot line or the 3.66 meter line. The time of the faster of two walks was used for scoring. Refer to Figure 4.41. Calculate the score for the walk test using these criteria.

Walk Test: Gait Ordinal Score
0 = could not do
1 = > 5.7 seconds (< 0.43 meters/ seconds)
2 = 4.1 - 5.6 seconds (0.44-0.60 meters/ seconds)
3 = 3.2 − 4.0 seconds (0.61-0.77 meters/ seconds)
4 = < 3.1 seconds (> 0.78 meters/ seconds)

Repeated Chair Stand Test
Select a sturdy straight back chair without arm rests. Place the chair with a wall behind it for safety. Instruct the patient to fold his/her arms across the chest and to stand up from

a sitting position five times without stopping between chair stands. Ask the patient to perform the chair stand test as quickly as possible. Refer to Figure 4.42.

Begin the stopwatch when the patient begins to stand up. Count aloud each time the patient arises. Stop the stopwatch when the subject has straightened up completely for the fifth time. Also stop if the patient uses arms to stand, after 2 minutes if the patient has not completed 5 rises or if there is concern about the patient's safety. Have a person ready to catch the patient should he/she lose balance. Allow the patient to stop and rest if he/she becomes tired. The time keeps going for a maximum of 2 minutes.

Record the number of chair stands completed and the total time in seconds if 5 stands are completed. Watch for the presence of imbalance. Calculate chair stand ordinal score for completing 5 chair stands using these criteria.

Chair Stand Ordinal Score
1 = >16.7 seconds
2 = 13.7 to 16.6 seconds
3 = 11.2 to 13.6 seconds
4 = <11.1 seconds

Standing Balance
Standing balance tests requires a patient to stand on 3 different foot positions of increasing difficulty without an assistive device. These tests should be carried out in bare feet.

Describe and demonstrate each test to the patient. Stand by the patient to assist in assuming the proper position. Allow the patient to hold on to the assessors arm to get balanced before starting the test. Ask the patient to indicate when he/she is ready to begin the test unaided. Timing is stopped if the person moves his/her feet from the proper position or the assessor provides contact to prevent a fall or the person touches the wall or other support surface with a hand. Inability to assume or maintain that position is equivalent to a failed test score. Have a sturdy chair nearby for support if needed.

Start with the easiest test first. The patient is asked to attempt to maintain his/her feet in the side-by-side position and hold this position for 10 seconds without holding on to a support surface or assistive device. Record the number of seconds for the side by side position and note the presence of imbalance.

The next level of difficulty is the semi-tandem stand in which the heel of one foot is beside the big toe of the other foot. Allow the patient to choose which foot is placed in front. The patient may need to hold on to the assessor's arm to gain balance before the test begins. Record the number of seconds for the standing semi-tandem position and note the presence of imbalance. Refer to Figure 4. 43.

The tandem stand is the most difficult of this battery of tests. It requires the patient to place the heel of one foot directly in front of the other foot and hold the position for 10 seconds. Allow the patient to choose which foot is placed in front. The patient may need to hold on to the assessor's arm to gain balance before the test begins. Record the number of seconds for the standing tandem position and note the presence of imbalance. Refer to Figure 4. 44. Calculate standing balance ordinal score using these criteria.

Standing Balance Ordinal Score

1 = side-by-side standing position for 10 seconds, but were unable to hold a semi-tandem position for 10 seconds

2 = hold a semi-tandem position for 10 seconds and full tandem position 0-2 seconds

3 = hold a semi-tandem position for 10 seconds and full tandem position for 3 to 9 seconds

4 = hold full tandem position for 10 seconds

Interpreting Measures of Lower Extremity Physical Function & Performance

Sum the performance scores for the tests of walking, repeatedly rising from a chair, and standing balance. The range of scores will be from 0 = worst performance to 12 = best performance. The validity of this scale has been demonstrated in analyses showing a gradient of risk of admission to a nursing home and mortality along the full range of the scale. Failure to complete one or more of these tests indicates deficits in strength and balance. More research is needed to correlate findings with changes in muscle mass and nutrition status (Guralnik, 1994, 1995; Ha, 2010; Gardner, 2001).

Example 4.4

Mrs. R, 70 yr F, 60 in., 91 lbs., lives at Star County Nursing Center. She had a CVA 2 months ago. With extensive rehabilitation, she has made great strides in increasing her lower body strength. Calculate her performance scores for the tests of walking, standing balance, and repeatedly rising from a chair.

Walk test: 4.5 sec to walk 8 feet
Balance test: semi-tandem position held for 10 seconds, tandem position held for 5 seconds
Chair Stand: 4 chair stands in 2 minutes

Answer: Refer to end of chapter.

Resistance Muscle Testing

During the assessment of the extremities, observe for bilateral symmetry, edema, presence of trauma and other abnormalities. Check the tonicity of muscle by asking the patient to squeeze examiner's fingers and noting for equality of contraction. Perform range of motion and test for muscle strength. Muscle strength can be evaluated against gravity and against resistance. Refer to Figures 4.45-4.48.

The purpose of resistance muscle testing is to determine the extent of muscular weakness as the result of an injury, disease or disuse. Anti-gravity resistive muscle testing was first developed by Dr. Robert Lovett, Professor of Orthopedic Surgery at Harvard Medical School, in 1912. The principle of resistive muscle testing is to isolate each muscle and apply a resistive force against the muscle as it moves your limb against gravity. Table 4.7. notes the Lovett scale for grading muscle strength and functional level. This tool may be useful in assessing improvement in muscle strength following MNT. More research is needed to correlate findings with improvement in nutrition status.

Table 4.7. Lovett Scale for Muscle Strength & Functional Level

Functional Level	Lovett Scale	Grade	% of Normal
No evidence of contractility	Zero (Z)	0	0
Evidence of slight contractility	Trace (T)	1	10
Complete ROM without gravity	Poor (P)	2	25
Complete ROM with gravity	Fair (F)	3	50
Complete ROM against gravity with some resistance	Good (G)	4	75
Complete ROM against gravity with full resistance	Normal (N)	5	100

(Lovett, 1916)

Eating Disorders

Malnutrition, diminished strength and function are often seen with eating disorders. The characteristics of malnutrition and measures of functional strength may be useful in assessing this population. Every patient with an eating disorder presents a unique set of characteristics. The RDN has to determine the nutrition diagnoses and recommend appropriate interventions based on the individual's specific situation. Generally speaking, an eating disorder is marked by extremes. It is present when a person experiences severe disturbances in eating behavior, such as extreme reduction of food intake or extreme overeating, feelings of extreme distress or concern about body weight or shape. Types of eating disorders include anorexia nervosa, bulimia nervosa, binge-eating disorder and eating disorders not otherwise specified (EDNOS).

Anorexia nervosa is characterized by emaciation, intense fear of gaining weight, relentless pursuit of thinness and unwillingness to maintain a healthy weight. These patients often have a distorted body image, a self-esteem that is heavily influenced by perceptions of body weight and shape, and a denial of the seriousness of low body weight. Bulimia nervosa is characterized by recurrent and frequent episodes of eating large amounts of food and feeling a lack of control over these episodes. Binge-eating is followed by behavior that compensates for the overeating such as forced vomiting, excessive use of laxatives or diuretics, fasting, excessive exercise, or a combination of these behaviors.

Individuals with bulimia nervosa usually maintain a healthy weight, while some are slightly overweight. They often fear gaining weight, want desperately to lose weight, and are intensely unhappy with their body size and shape.

Usually, bulimic behavior is done secretly several times a week to many times a day. Individuals with binge-eating disorder lose control over eating and are often overweight or obese. Unlike bulimia nervosa, episodes of binge-eating are not followed by purging, excessive exercise or fasting.

Practical Applications for NFPA: Eating Disorders
Signs of eating disorders develop insidiously. Hallmarks of anorexia nervosa that may be identified through a review of the medical history include osteopenia or osteoporosis, mild anemia, severe constipation, hypotension, decreased body temperature and infertility. Patients may report lethargy or sluggishness. Using NFPA, the clinician may observe brittle hair and nails, dry, yellowish skin, lanugo (growth of fine hair all over the body, Figure 4.49), mild muscle wasting and weakness, slowed breathing and pulse, delayed growth and development and amenorrhea in girls and women.

Signs of bulimia nervosa that may be identified through a medical history review include chronically inflamed or sore throat, swollen salivary gland in neck and jaw, worn tooth enamel, GERD, laxative abuse, and abnormal lab test results suggesting electrolyte imbalance or dehydration. Using NFPA, the RDN may observe Russell's Sign (scraped or raw areas on the patient's knuckles caused by self-induced vomiting) in those who purge using vomiting. Refer to Figure 4.50. Absence of this sign is not an indication of the absence of purging. Patients may use foreign objects such as tooth brush heads or straws to induce vomiting (Wilson, 2005; Steinhausen, 2008).

Nutrition diagnoses that may apply include suboptimal nutrient intake or macro and micronutrients, underweight, altered nutrition-related lab test results, harmful beliefs about food, disordered eating pattern and excessive physical activity. Figures 4.1-4.6 are examples of changes in body composition due to fat loss that reflect either non-severe or severe malnutrition.

Figure 4.1. Orbital

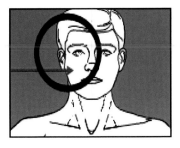

Figure 4.2. Orbital Fat Loss

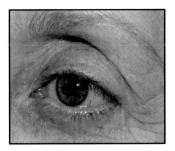

Figure 4.3. Buccal Fat

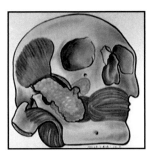

Figure 4.4. Buccal Fat Loss

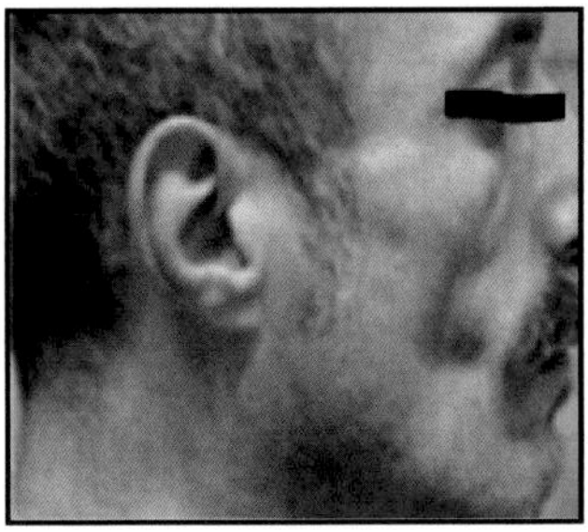

Figure 4.5. Facial Fat Loss

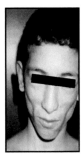

Figure 4.6. Fat Loss Over Ribs

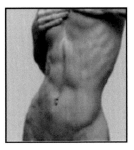

Figures 4.7-4.33 are examples of changes in body composition due to fat and muscle loss that reflect either non-severe or severe malnutrition.

Figures 4.7.-4.8. Severe Fat and Muscle Wasting

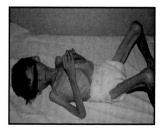 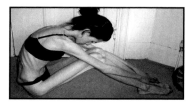

Figure 4.9. Triceps   **Figure 4.10.** Fat Loss Overlying Triceps

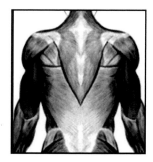 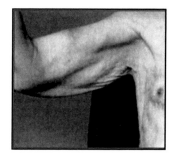

Figure 4.11. Temporalis   **Figure 4.12.** Temporal Wasting

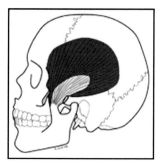 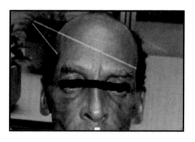

Figure 4.13. Interosseous **Figure 4.14.** Normal vs. Wasting

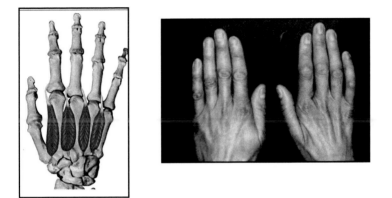

Figures 4.15.-4.17. Upper Body: Biceps, Deltoid, Trapezius

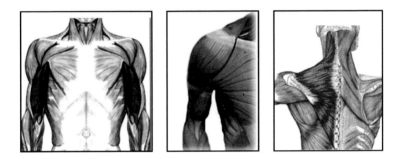

Figures 4.18.-4.19. Latissimus Dorsi

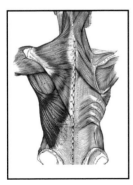
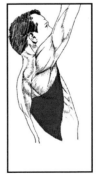

Figures 4.20-4.21. Upper Body Wasting

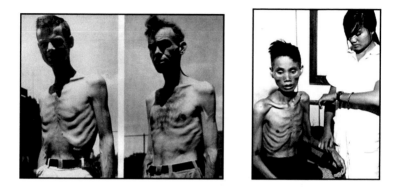

Figures 4.22.-4.23. Acromion Process

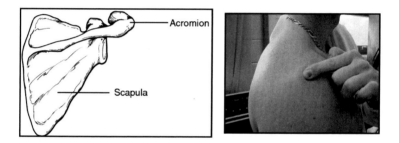

Figure 4.24. Scapula Wasting   **Figure 4.25.** Trapezius Wasting

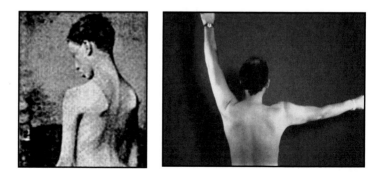

Figures 4.26.-4.27. Lower Body: Quadriceps, Gastrocnemius

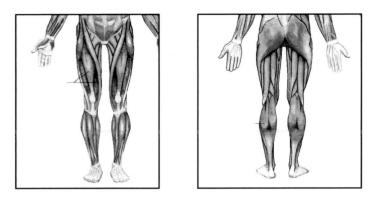

Figures 4.28.-4.29. Quadricep Wasting

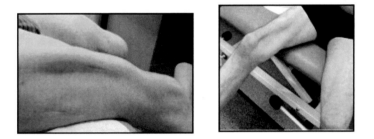

Figure 4.30. Muscle Wasting **Figure 4.31.** Unilateral Wasting

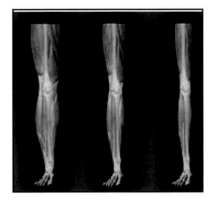
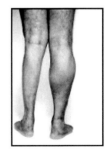

Figures 4.32.-4.33. Pitting Edema

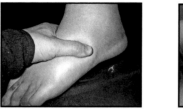 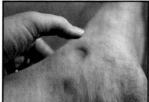

Figure 4.34. Non-Pitting Edema

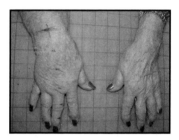

Figures 4.35.-4.38. Degrees of Edema; 1+, 2+, 3+, 4+

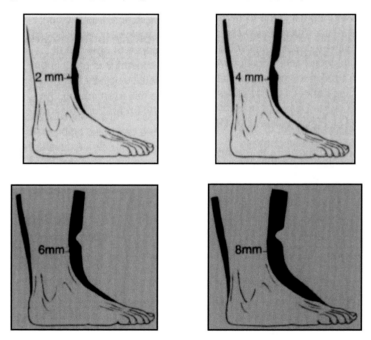

Figures 4.39.-4.45. illustrate measures of physical function and performance.

Figure 4.39. Dynamometer   **Figure 4.40.** Hand Grip Strength

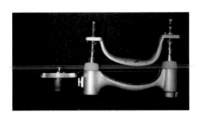
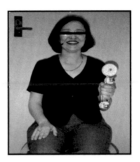

Figure 4.41. Walk Test   **Figure 4.42.** Chair Stand Test

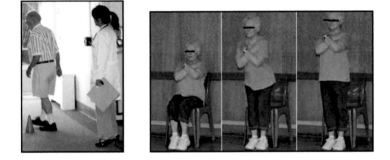

Figures 4.43.-4.44. Standing Balance: Semi-tandem, Tandem

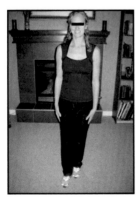
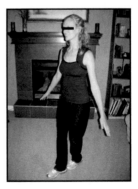

Figures 4.45.-4.48. Measures of Diminished Strength

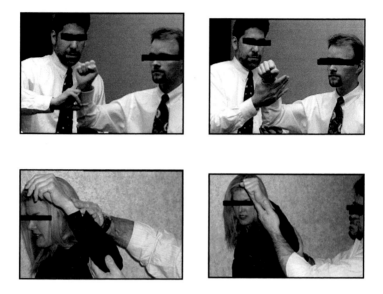

Figures 4.49.-4.50. illustrate signs of eating disorders.

Figure 4.49. Lanugo   **Figure 4.50. Russell's Sign**

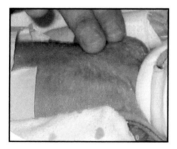

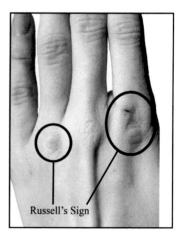

Russell's Sign

Key: Examples in Chapter 4

4.1. Using the Mifflin-St. Jeor Equation, her estimated total energy expenditure is about 800 Kcal/d. If she is eating half of the meal served, she is consuming about 1000 calories or about 200 Kcal more than her estimated needs. She does not meet the criteria for reduced dietary intake.

4.2. Using her Usual wt 90 lbs - 80 = 10 lbs loss or 11 % loss. Using her hospital discharge wt 85-80 = 5 lbs. or 5.9% loss. Her weight loss meets the criteria for unintended weight loss.

4.3. Yes, she has one or more areas of muscle wasting.

4.4. Walk test: 4 seconds to walk 8 feet

Score = 3

Balance test: semi-tandem position held for 10 seconds, tandem position held for 5 seconds

Score = 3

Chair Stand: 3 chair stands in 2 minutes

Score = zero. 5 chair stands are required to receive points

Total score= 6 out a maximum of 12 points

References

American Dietetic Association. Nutrition Care Manual. Characteristics of Malnutrition. Chicago, IL: ADA, 2011.

Bauer, J, Kaiser, M (2008) Mini Nutritional Assessment- its history, today's practice & future perspectives. Nutr Clin Prac. 23:388-396.

Becker AE, Grinspoon SK, Klibanski A. Eating disorders. New England Journal of Medicine, 1999; 340(14):1092–1098.

Blackburn,GL Bistrian,B Nutritional and metabolic assessment of the hospitalized patient. JPEN 1977,1:11-22.

Bohannon, R (2010) Grip strength impairments among older adults receiving physical therapy in a home care setting. Perceptual and Motor Skills: 111(3) 761-764.

CMS: MDS 3.0 for Nursing Home. http://www.cms.gov/NursingHomeQualityInits/30_NHQIMDS30TechnicalInformation.asp#Top OfPage.htm. Accessed November 17, 2011.

Cooper, B (2002) validity of subjective global assessment as a nutritional marker in end stage renal disease. A JKD 40(1) 126-132.

Covinsky, KE (2002) Malnutrition and bad outcomes J Gen Intern Med 17(12) 956-7.

Covinsky, KE, Martin, GE, (1999). The relationship between clinical assessment of nutritional status and adverse outcomes in older hospitalized medical patients. JAGS 47(5) 532-8.

Cuthbert,S, Goodheart,G On the reliability and validity of manual muscle testing: a literature review. Chirorp Osteopat 2007 15:4

Ferguson M et al. (1999) Development of a valid and reliable malnutrition screening tool for adult acute hospital patients. Nutrition 15, (6): 458-464.

Gardner,M, Buchner,D Practical implementation of an exercise-based falls prevention program. J Age & Ageing 2001: 30: 77-83

Guralnik , JM, Ferrucci , L. Lower-Extremity Function in Persons over the Age of 70 Years as a Predictor of Subsequent Disability. N Engl J Med 1995; 332:556-562.

Guralnik JM, Simonsick EM, Ferrucci L, et al. A short physical performance battery assessing lower extremity function: association with self-reported disability and prediction of mortality and nursing home admission. J Gerontol 1994;49:M85-M94

Ha L, Hauge T, Spenning A. Individual, nutritional support prevents undernutrition, increases muscle strength and improves QoL among elderly at nutritional risk hospitalized for acute stroke: a randomized, controlled trial. Clin Nutr. 2010.29(5). 567-573.

Hagan, JC. Acute and chronic diseases. In Mulner, RM, ed. Encyclopedia of Health Services Research. vol 1. Thousand Oaks, CA:Sage; 2009:25.

Humphreys J, de la MP, Hirsch S, Barrera G, Gattas V, Bunout D. Muscle strength as a predictor of loss of functional status in hospitalized patients. Nutrition. 2002;18:616–620

Jensen GL, Hsiao PY.(2010) Obesity in older adults: Relationship to functional limitation. Current Opinion Clinical Nutrition and Metabolic Care, 13: 46-51.

Jensen, G, Bistrian, B (2009) Malnutrition syndromes: a conundrum vs continuum JPEN 33(6) 710-716.

Jensen, G, Mirtallo,J (2010) Adult starvation and disease-related malnutrition: a proposal for etiology-based diagnosis in the clinical practice setting from the International Consensus Guideline Committee. JPEN 34(2) 156-159.

Kaburagi, T, Hirasawa (2011) Nutritional status is strongly correlated with grip strength and depression in community-living elderly Japanese. Public Health Nutrition. DOI: 10.1017/S1368980011000346.

Kaiser MJ, Bauer JM, Rämsch C, et al. (2010) Frequency of Malnutrition in Older Adults: A Multinational Perspective Using the Mini Nutritional Assessment. J Am Geriatr Soc 58 (9) 1734-8.

Kaiser R. Functionality & mortality in obese nursing home residents: example of risk factor paradox? JAMDA 2010;11(6):428-435.

Kaiser, MJ, Bauer, C (2009)Validation of the Mini Nutritional Assessment short form (MNA®-SF): A Practical tool for identification of nutritional status. J Nutrition, Health & Aging 13 (9).

Kaur, N, Koley, S (2010) An Association of Nutritional Status and Hand Grip Strength in Female Laborers of North India. Anthropologist 12(4)237-243.

Keys, A chronic undernutrition and starvation with notes on protein deficiency. JAMA. 1948: 138: 500-511.

Klein, S, Kinney, J Nutrition support in clinical practice: review of published data and recommendations for future research directions. NIH, ASPEN, ASCN. JPEN 1977: 21: 133-156.

Lovett RW, Martin EG. Certain aspects of infantile paralysis with a description of a method of muscle testing. JAMA. 1916, Mar 4, 729–33.

Norman, K . Hand grip strength: Outcome predictor and marker of nutritional status. Clin Nutr 2011:30:135-142.

Norman K, Three month intervention with protein & energy rich supplements improves muscle function & quality of life in malnourished patients with non-neoplastic gastrointestinal disease – a randomized controlled trial. Clin Nutr. 2008;27:48–56

Norman K, Schutz T, Kemps M, Josef LH, Lochs H, Pirlich M. The Subjective Global Assessment reliably identifies malnutrition-related muscle dysfunction. Clin Nutr. 2005;24:143–150

Norman, K, (2011) Hand grip strength: outcome predictor and marker of nutritional status. Clinical Nutrition 30(2) 135-142.

Nursal, T, Noyan, T (2005) Simple two-part tool for screening of malnutrition. Nutrition 21(6) 659-665.

Pieterse, S, Manandhar, M (2002) The association between nutritional status and handgrip strength in older Rwandan refugees EJCN 56(10) 933-939.

Rossiter-Fornoff, JE, Wolf, SL et al A cross-sectional validation study of the FICSIT common data base static balance measures. J Gerontol Med Sci 1995, 50 A: M291-7

Soeters, P, (2009) Advances in understanding and assessing malnutrition. Current Opinions in Clin Nutr Metab Care 12: 487-494.

Steinhausen HC. Outcomes of eating disorders. Child and Adolescent Psychiatric Clinics of North America, 2008; 18:225–242.

Wang, A, Sea, M (2005)Evaluation of handgrip strength as a nutritional marker and prognostic indicator in peritoneal dialysis patients. AJCN 81(1) 79-86.

Wilson GT and Shafran R. Eating disorders guidelines from NICE. Lancet, 2005; 365:79–81.

Chapter 5
Tools for Assessing Skin, Hair & Nails

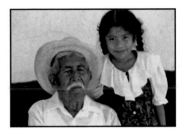

During a general survey of overall appearance, observe the skin on the face, arms and hands, nails and hair. The characteristics the RDN is looking for are signs that might suggest a nutrient deficiency or toxicity. Patients often notice changes in their skin, hair or nails before the clinician does. Some questions to consider include:

Skin:
- Have you noticed any changes in your skin?
- Does the skin have an increased (brownness) or decreased pigmentation?
- Does the skin have a red cast or tone?
- Does the skin have a blue cast or tone?
- Does the skin have a yellow cast or tone?

Figure 5.1. Follicular Hyperkeratosis (Vitamin A deficiency)

Figure 5.2. Pellagra (Niacin deficiency)

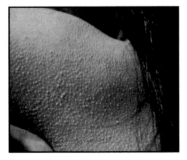

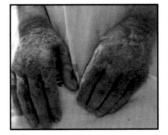

- Evaluate the moisture of the skin.
- Does the skin look dry and scaly, or sweaty or oily?
- Is the skin warm or cold to the touch?
- Is the skin rough or smooth?
- Are there lesions or rash on the skin?
- Does the patient have acute surgical wounds?
- Does the patient have a history or skin breakdown?
- Does the patient have nutrition risk factors for skin breakdown such as low BMI, unplanned weight loss, low nutrient density intake?
- Is the patient at increased risk for prolonged pressure on bony prominences or other areas of the skin?
- Does the patient have skin breakdown?

Figure 5.3. Anatomy of Skin

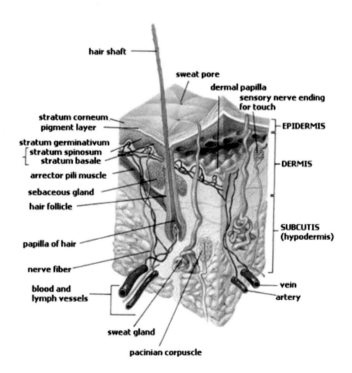

The skin is the largest organ in the body that contributes about 10 percent of the total body weight. The skin is a bilayered organ that serves as the first line of defense against a variety of assaults. The epidermis is the thin outer layer and the dermis is the thicker inner layer.

Skin changes over time with age, exposure to sun, hydration, medications and nutrition. It is often ignored until it is injured. Skin and nails are thinner at birth, increase in density through adolescence. Once adulthood is reached, the dermis decreases in thickness by about 20 percent, but the epidermis is about the same thickness. However, the epidermal turnover time increases making wound healing a longer process. In young adults the epidermal turnover is about 21 days, however, by age 35 the turnover time is more than 40 days.

The skin of an older adult is more easily injured due to changes in the epidermal-dermal junctions. Skin elasticity also decreases with age. Collagen fibers appear to unwind and elastin fibers breakdown. The degradation of elastin begins to occur around age 30, but is markedly observed by age 70 (Braverman, 1986).

The barrier function of the skin decreases with age making skin irritations more common. Protection against ultraviolet radiation is diminished with age due to a reduced number of melanocytes which in turn contributes to wrinkling and sagging skin. The sagging is due in part to the loss of underlying tissue and the loss of elastin and collagen. Wrinkles are due to an increase in dryness of the skin.

The sensory receptors in the skin are diminished in capacity with aging. The risk of being burned or injured is more common due to a decreased sensation. Vitamin D production in the skin decreases with age and supplementation of vitamin D may be necessary for individuals with limited exposure to sunlight.

Nutrient deficiencies and toxicities can result in changes in skin color and texture and changes in the mucous membranes. While nutrient deficiencies are rare, these are reported in adults with malabsorptive disorders and following weight loss surgery. Toxicities are reported in individuals taking megadoses of vitamin mineral supplements.

Numerous medications affect the skin as noted on Table 5.1 (Potts, 1990). Corticosteroids are known to interfere with epidermal regeneration and collagen synthesis (Ehrlich, 1968).

Table 5.1. Categories of Medications that can Affect Skin

• Analgesics	• Diuretics
• Antibacterials	• Hypoglycemic agents
• Antihypertensives	• Oral contraceptives
• Antihistamines	• Sunscreens
• Antineoplastic agents	• Tricyclic antidepressants
• Antipsychotic agents	

Skin & Nutrient Deficiencies

The skin color, texture, dryness, temperature, abnormal mucous membranes and presence of lesions or injuries are all characteristics to note in NFPA. Abnormalities should be corroborated with data from lab test results, anthropometric data, dietary history, vital signs and other clinical assessment data noted by the other medical team members

Review the medical history for contributors to impaired nutrient utilization.

Practical Applications for NFPA: Color

The color of normal skin depends primarily on four pigments as noted in Table 5.2.

Table 5.2. Skin Pigments

Pigments	Color
Melanin	Brown
Carotene	Golden yellow
Oxyhemoglobin	Bright red
Deoxyhemoglobin	Blue

Changes in skin color may also be due to a number of medical conditions. Inspect the skin for abnormal color. Compare the findings to other evidence in the medical records that suggest a change in medical condition or functional status. The nutrition professional is looking for changes that suggest impaired ability to prepare meals, impaired functional status to eat, nutrient deficiency or nutrient overload.

Increased Brownness of Skin

The amount of melanin in the skin is genetically determined. It can also be increased with exposure to sunlight. Individuals with areas of darker, thick, velvety skin in body folds and creases may have acanthosis nigricans. It is more often seen in patients of African and Hispanic/ Latino descent. Acanthosis nigricans usually appears slowly and doesn't cause any symptoms other than skin changes. It results in velvety light-brown to black markings in body creases such as in the armpits, neck folds, and over the joints of the fingers and toes. Refer to Figures 5.4.-5.6.

Acanthosis nigricans is seen in patients with obesity, insulin resistance, metabolic syndrome, hypertension, dyslipidemia, Addison's disease, disorders of pituitary gland, hypothyroidism and growth hormone therapy. It has been shown to be a reliable early marker for metabolic syndrome in children (Otto, 2010).

Weight management and improved glucose control can help prevent acanthosis nigricans as well as improve medical management of endocrine disorders (Kong, 2010). Patients with lymphoma, cancers of the gastrointestinal or genitourinary tracts can also develop severe cases of acanthosis nigricans.

Occasionally acanthosis nigricans is medication-induced. Medications associated with acanthosis nigricans, include nicotinic acid, insulin, pituitary extract, systemic corticosteroids, diethylstilbestrol, triazinate, oral contraceptives, fusidic acid, and methyltestosterone (Miller, 2011, Otto, 2010).

Increased Yellow Cast to Skin

Jaundice or icterus occurs when excess amounts of serum bilirubin dissolve in the subcutaneous fat, causing a yellowish appearance of the skin and the whites of the eyes. The yellowing may extend to other tissues and body fluids as well as turn the urine a darker color. Jaundice is not a disease, but a sign of a variety of medical conditions. It can occur when the normal process of destruction of red blood cells and elimination of bilirubin is interrupted. This occurs when there is excessive hemolysis, liver disease that reduces the ability of the liver to remove and modify bilirubin, or obstruction to the flow of bile into the intestine (Bickley, 2009). Refer to Figure 5.7.

A lemon-yellow–tinged pallor to the skin is reported in pernicious anemia. Other physical signs and symptoms include raw-beefy red tongue lacking filiform papillae, paresthesia (sensation of pins and needles) in extremities, loss of sense of touch, changes in gait, stiffness in arms and legs, dementia, hallucinations and paranoia (Bickley, 2009). Refer to Figure 5.15 and Chapter 9.

Increased Yellow to Orange Cast to Skin

Carotene exists in subcutaneous fat. Hypercarotenemia or carotenemia is characterized by a yellow to orange skin color. It is due to consuming too much beta carotene supplements or eating too many dietary sources of beta carotene, (orange juice, carrots, carrot juice or pumpkin) In hypercarotenemia, the whites of the eyes remain white, unlike jaundice who have a yellowish tinge to the eyes (Schwartz, 2011). Refer to Figure 5.8.

Increased Bluish Cast of Skin

The form of hemoglobin that circulates without oxygen is called deoxyhemoglobin. Increased concentration in cutaneous blood vessels gives skin a bluish cast called cyanosis. There are two forms of cyanosis. If the arterial blood oxygen level is low, cyanosis is central. Central cyanosis is best identified in the lips, oral mucosa and tongue. In dark skinned individuals, look at the palms, nails and soles of feet. If the arterial blood oxygen level is normal, cyanosis is peripheral. Peripheral cyanosis occurs when the cutaneous blood flow decreases or slows and tissues extract more oxygen than usual from the blood. It is a normal response to anxiety or a cold environment.

Cyanosis that is seen in only one part of the body may be due to a blood clot. It is often seen in patients with chronic heart or lung problems (Bickley, 2009). Refer to Figure 5.9.

Decreased Color of Skin

The form of hemoglobin that circulates carrying oxygen is called oxyhemoglobin. Very pale skin or pallor and pale conjunctivae suggest a lack of oxygen possibly due to a nutritional anemia. See anemia section. Refer to Figures 5.10.-5.11.

Increased Redness of Skin

An increased redness of skin is caused by an increase in blood flow through the arteries to the capillaries causing a reddening of the skin. Blushing is a normal body response to strong emotion. Flushing of the face may be related to high fever, menopause, hyperthyroidism, rosacea, intense exercise, spicy foods, caffeine, niacin supplements, or medications. Increased erythema in other parts of the body may suggest inflammation, tissue injury, rash, skin disorder or infection (Bickley, 2009).

Clinical Nutrition Pearls: Skin Color

Diseases and disorders associated with changes in skin are medical diagnoses. The nutrition professional is identifying nutrition diagnoses. PES statements may incorporate NFPA observations specific to skin color, medical signs and symptoms related to changes in skin color, dietary data and anthropometric data. Nutrition diagnoses that may apply include altered nutrition-related lab test results, excessive or suboptimal intake of micro or macronutrients, excessive bioactive substance intake or harmful beliefs about food. Use NFPA findings as a benchmark to monitor and evaluate effectiveness of nutrition interventions.

Practical Applications for NFPA:
Nutritional Anemias

Anemia is symptomatic of a disease and is a biomarker for increased morbidity, hospitalizations, mortality and increased healthcare costs. The prevalence of anemia increases with each decade of life over age 70 and is associated with both frailty and mobility impairment (AMDA, 2007).

A very pale skin color and pale conjunctivae are two signs of anemia. Anemia may be caused by acute or chronic blood loss, deficient erythropoiesis, or excessive hemolysis. There are four common types of nutrition related anemias;
- iron deficiency anemia
- pernicious anemia
- megaloblastic anemia
- anemia of chronic and inflammatory diseases

Other rare types of nutritional anemias include vitamin B_6 deficiency, an overload of zinc resulting in a copper deficiency or lead toxicity causing iron deficiency anemia.

Common symptoms of nutritional anemias include fatigue, unusually rapid heart rate, shortness of breath with exercise, difficulty concentrating, dizziness, leg cramps and insomnia. Individuals with iron deficiency may also have pica, soreness of the mouth with stomatitis and koilonychia (spooned nails). Iron deficiency anemia results from insufficient dietary intake or impaired utilization or a combination of factors (Santo, 1991).

Physical signs uniquely associated with pernicious anemia include lemon-yellow–tinged pallor with raw-beefy red tongue lacking filiform papillae (Figure 5.15), paresthesia in extremities, loss of sense of touch, changes in gait, stiffness in arms and legs, dementia, hallucinations and paranoia. Pernicious anemia results from insufficient dietary intake of vitamin B12 or impaired utilization of vitamin B12 or insufficient intrinsic factor required for absorption or a combination of factors.

Individuals with megaloblastic anemia may have increased weakness, impaired cognitive function, irritability and anorexia. Megaloblastic anemia results from insufficient dietary intake of folate or impaired utilization of folate or a combination of factors.

Individuals with anemias caused by inflammatory and chronic diseases may also complain of syncope, palpitations, cold intolerance, and anorexia. Chronic diseases associated with anemias include congestive heart failure, chronic kidney disease and other inflammatory disorders that result in redistribution of iron stores and poor iron utilization.

Vitamin B_6 deficiency contributes to an impaired transsulfuration of methionine to cysteine resulting in elevated levels of homocysteine. It is also required to convert folate into its active form for DNA synthesis. Vitamin B_6 deficiency is rare, but may be secondary to malnutrition, malabsorption, sickle cell anemia, alcoholism or use of pyridoxine-inactivating medications (i.e. anticonvulsants, isoniazid, cycloserine, hydralazine, corticosteroids and penicillamine). It is associated with microcytic anemia, dermatitis with cheilosis and glossitis, pellagra-like syndrome, peripheral neuropathy depression and confusion, and weakened immune function.

Signs and symptoms of anemia caused by lead poisoning

include a blue-black line on the gums (Figure 5.17. lead line), abdominal pain, constipation, nausea, vomiting changes in mood, peripheral neuropathy, memory loss and encephalopathy. Lead interferes with iron utilization and dietary supplements are ineffective (Bickley, 2009).

Copper deficiencies are rare, but can be the result of zinc overload or malabsorption. Cooper deficiencies have been reported in individuals following malabsorptive weight loss surgeries. Physical signs of a copper deficiency include numbness in lower extremities, abnormal gait, myelopathy, poor wound healing or dehiscence of wounds. Copper related anemia does not respond to iron or vitamin B12 supplementation.

When an anemia is suspected, look for other corroborating evidence in the medical record or from the interview. Review lab reports for abnormal test results for hemoglobin, hematocrit, serum iron, ferritin and MVC. Determine if the anemia is microcytic, normocytic or macrocytic. If labs suggest macrocytic anemias or vitamin B12 deficiency, additional tests are needed including serum vitamin B12, methylmalonic, acid and folate. Review medications for folate antagonists.

For individuals with suspected lead-poisoning, review lab reports for abnormal test results for hemoglobin, hematocrit, serum iron and ferritin since lead interferes with the absorption of iron. Follow up testing is needed for confirmation to include lead levels and zinc protoporphyrin.

Abnormal labs reported in copper-related anemia include very low hemoglobin, hematocrit and leukocytes. However, MCV, vitamin B12, folate, ferritin and platelet count are usually within normal ranges. **Figures 5.11-5.18** are examples of physical signs associated with nutritional anemias.

Figures 5.4.-5.6. Acanthosis Nigricans

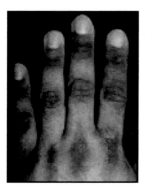

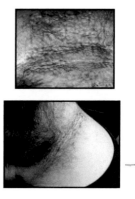

Figure 5.7. Jaundice

Figure 5.8. Hypercarotenemia

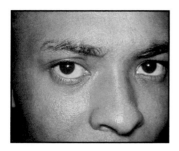

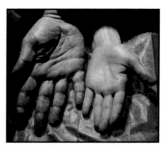

Figure 5.9. Cyanosis

Figure 5.10. Pallor

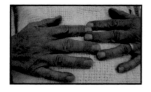

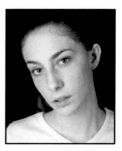

Figure 5.11. Pale Conjunctivae **Figure 5.12.** Stomatitis

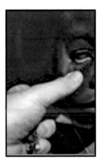 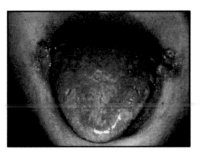

Figure 5.13. Koilonychia **Figure 5.14.** Beefy-Red Tongue

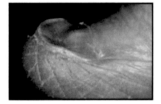 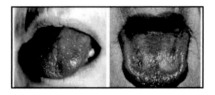

Figure 5.15. Lemon-yellow Pallor with Slick Tongue **Figure 5.16.** Slick Tongue

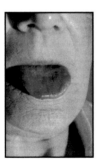 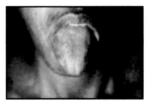

Figure 5.17. Lead Line **Figure 5.18.** Wound Dehiscence

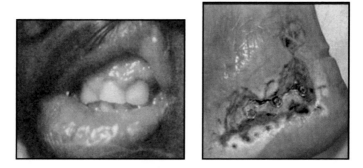

Clinical Nutrition Pearls: Anemia

Diseases and disorders associated with nutritional anemias are medical diagnoses. Nutrition diagnoses that may apply include altered nutrition-related lab test results, excessive or suboptimal intake of micro or macronutrients, excessive bioactive substance intake or harmful beliefs about food. Use NFPA findings as a benchmark to gauge improvement in nutrition status.

Risk Assessment & Etiology of Skin Failure

Normal healthy skin can be damaged by mechanical and chemical assaults, poor vascularization and infections. With aging, the skin becomes more fragile. Poor nutrition compounds the problem and may contribute to slow wound healing and increased risk for skin damage. Once the skin is broken, both intrinsic and systemic factors will impede the normal cascade of healing (Litchford, 2010).

There are many different types of wounds seen in healthcare settings including surgical wounds, trauma wounds and skin breakdown. The AMDA Clinical Practice Guideline, Pressure Ulcers in the Long Term Care Setting (2008) categorizes

skin breakdown into four groups:
- Pressure ulcers
- Diabetic ulcers
- Ischemic ulcers
- Venous ulcers

Not all wounds respond to the same treatment. Some wounds will heal quickly, while others may take a long time to heal. A few wounds will never heal. All types of skin breakdown require special attention and care. Intervention strategies need to be consistent with the clinical goals of the patient/resident and the family.

Practical Applications for NFPA: Skin

Pressure ulcers are the most common type of skin breakdown seen in adults. These wounds are caused by a combination of factors including increased pressure on a bony prominence and poor nutrition status.

Poor nutrition is not always present in patients with pressure ulcers, but adequate nutrients are required for healing. Patients entering an acute care setting may not be at nutrition risk for skin breakdown upon admission, but may be at risk after lengthy surgeries, after extended stays in ICU or after being bedbound on a standard mattress.

The National Pressure Ulcer Advisory Panel (NPUAP, 2010) published risk assessment criteria, guidelines for preventing pressure ulcers, staging criteria for pressure ulcers and guidelines for treatment of skin breakdown. In addition, they have specific nutrition recommendations for prevention and for treatment of pressure ulcers. Refer to Resources section at the end of this chapter for more detailed information on the skin assessment.

Start the skin risk assessment by gathering data from the

medical record. Aspects of nutrition status associated with an increased risk for skin breakdown include:

- Reduced body mass index (BMI)
- Low body weight
- Low dietary intake of protein
- Low serum albumin and prealbumin (suggesting inflammatory processes)
- Hypocholesterolemia
- Decreased total lymphocyte count (suggesting compromised immune response)
- Nutritional anemias
- Altered ability to self-feed
- Reduced food intake (Horn, 2002; Lyder, 2001; Selvaag, 2002; Consortium for Spinal Cord Medicine, 2000)
- Requiring assistance with 7 or more ADLs (Horn, 2004)

If skin breakdown is already present, review the wound care nursing assessment and progress notes in addition to the nutrition risk assessment. Review lab test results for dehydration, nutritional anemias and poorly controlled chronic diseases. Review food and water intake data and compare to estimated requirements. Refer to NPUAP Guidelines for increased nutrient requirements for individuals at risk for skin breakdown and with skin breakdown (NPUAP, 2010).

Collaborate with the wound care nurse or treatment nurse to visually assess skin breakdown for the initial assessment and to monitor and evaluate healing. Always use standard and universal precautions to protect the patient and yourself from the spread of disease.

The NPUAP has established definitions for different stages of pressure ulcers. These definitions replace previous designations published by the AHCPR. Definitions are reprinted with permission from NPUAP.

Pressure Ulcer Definition

A pressure ulcer is localized injury to the skin and/or underlying tissue usually over a bony prominence, as a result of pressure, or pressure in combination with shear and/or friction. A number of contributing or confounding factors are also associated with pressure ulcers; the significance of these factors is yet to be elucidated.

Pressure Ulcer Stages: Suspected Deep Tissue Injury

Purple or maroon localized area of discolored intact skin or blood-filled blister due to damage of underlying soft tissue from pressure and/or shear. The area may be preceded by tissue that is painful, firm, mushy, boggy, warmer or cooler as compared to adjacent tissue. (Figure 5.22.)

Further Description:

Deep tissue injury may be difficult to detect in individuals with dark skin tones. Evolution may include a thin blister over a dark wound bed. The wound may further evolve and become covered by thin eschar. Evolution may be rapid exposing additional layers of tissue even with optimal treatment.

Pressure Ulcer Stages: Stage I

Intact skin with non-blanchable redness of a localized area usually over a bony prominence. Darkly pigmented skin may not have visible blanching; its color may differ from the surrounding area. (Note: blanching on pressure is fading of redness. This indicates that the color is probably due to dilatation of skin capillaries. Redness that is due to hemorrhage or abnormal pigmentation will not fade with pressure. Figure 5.23.)

Further Description:
The area may be painful, firm, soft, warmer or cooler as compared to adjacent tissue. Stage I may be difficult to detect in individuals with dark skin tones. May indicate "at risk" persons (a heralding sign of risk).

Pressure Ulcer Stages: Stage II
Partial thickness loss of dermis presenting as a shallow open ulcer with a red pink wound bed, without slough. May also present as an intact or open/ruptured serum-filled blister. (Figure 5.24.)

Further Description:
Presents as a shiny or dry shallow ulcer without slough or bruising. This stage should not be used to describe skin tears, tape burns, perineal dermatitis, maceration or excoriation. (Note:*Bruising indicates suspected deep tissue injury.)

Pressure Ulcer Stages: Stage III
Full thickness tissue loss. Subcutaneous fat may be visible but bone, tendon or muscle are not exposed. Slough may be present but does not obscure the depth of tissue loss. May include undermining and tunneling. (Figure 5.25.)

Further description:
The depth of a stage III pressure ulcer varies by anatomical location. The bridge of the nose, ear, occiput and malleolus do not have subcutaneous tissue and stage III ulcers can be shallow. In contrast, areas of significant adiposity can develop extremely deep stage III pressure ulcers. Bone/

tendon is not visible or directly palpable.

Pressure Ulcer Stages: Stage IV
Full thickness tissue loss with exposed bone, tendon or muscle. Slough or eschar may be present on some parts of the wound bed. Often include undermining and tunneling. (Figure 5.26.)

Further Description:
The depth of a stage IV pressure ulcer varies by anatomical location. The bridge of the nose, ear, occiput and malleolus do not have subcutaneous tissue and these ulcers can be shallow. Stage IV ulcers can extend into muscle and/or supporting structures (e.g., fascia, tendon or joint capsule) making osteomyelitis possible. Exposed bone/tendon is visible or directly palpable.

Pressure Ulcer Stages: Unstageable
Full thickness tissue loss in which the base of the ulcer is covered by slough (yellow, tan, gray, green or brown) and/or eschar (tan, brown or black) in the wound bed. (Figure 5.21.)

Further Description:
Until enough slough and/or eschar is removed to expose the base of the wound, the true depth, and therefore stage, cannot be determined. Stable (dry, adherent, intact without erythema or fluctuance) eschar on the heels serves as "the body's natural (biological) cover" and should not be removed.

Assessment for Signs of Healing
There are four stages of wound healing. Each stage is associated with key cellular interactions and clinical signs and symptoms as noted on Table 5.4 and illustrated on

Figures 5.27.-5.33. Collaborate with the wound care nurse to learn to recognize characteristics of each of the stages of pressure ulcers and to differentiate the different stages of wound healing. While the physician and wound care nurse will stage the wound and document changes in the wound, it is helpful for the RDN to be involved in the process. One indicator that nutrient needs are not being met is poor wound healing and wound dehiscence may be due to nutrient overload.

Chronic zinc supplementation can result in a copper deficiency since zinc, iron and copper all compete for the same receptor sites. One sign of a copper deficiency is dehiscence of a healed or healing wound. Work collaboratively with the wound care nurse for a global picture of the wound healing progress. Use NFPA data tosupport nutrition diagnoses and to serve as a benchmark for evaluating effectiveness of nutrition interventions.

Clinical Nutrition Pearls: Skin
The staging of wounds is a medical diagnosis. However the progress of the wound toward healing is done by an interdisciplinary team. Adequate nutrition is required for wounds to heal. One way to measure outcomes of nutrition interventions is to monitor wound healing. If the wound is not healing, the patient may require additional interventions that may include more energy, protein or selected micronutrients. Use of lab tests such as albumin and prealbumin provide little information on risk for skin breakdown or repletion of lean body mass (Litchford, 2011).

Nutrition diagnoses that may apply include excessive or suboptimal intake of micro or macronutrients, excessive alcohol intake, malnutrition, impaired nutrient utilization, swallowing or chewing difficulty, and unintended weight loss. Use NFPA findings as a benchmark to monitor and evaluate effectiveness of nutrition interventions.

Table 5.4. Stages of Wound Healing

Wound Healing Phase	Descriptor	Key Cellular Interactions	Clinical Signs & Symptoms
Hemostasis	Non-healing	Platelet activation, adhesion & aggregation; release of growth factors from platelets	Slowing of profuse bleeding; clot formation
Inflammation	Non-healing to early/partial granulation	Elevated neutrophils & cytokines. Macrophages secrete growth factors & cytokines; signal transition from inflammatory to proliferative phase	Inflamed area with slight induration & warmth around wound resolving
Proliferative	Early/partial granulation transitioning to fully granulating	Cell-cell & cell-matrix communication for synthesis & deposition of granulation tissue, ingrowth of new blood vessels; wound contraction & epithelization	Beefy red, slightly moist granulation; decreasing length, width & depth; pink epithelial tissue covers the wound
Remodeling	Fully granulating	Scar tissue transforms into stronger, more organized collagen bundles to improve tensile strength by cell-cell & cell-matrix interaction	Epithelial tissue turns from pink scar to translucent silver then white.

Figures 5.19-5.29. are examples of venous ulcers, pressure ulcers by stage and steps in wound healing.

Figures 5.19. Venous Ulcer

Figure 5.20. Slough

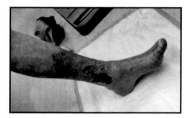

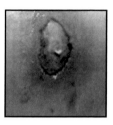

Figure 5.21. Unstageable Eschar

Figure 5.22. Deep Tissue Injury

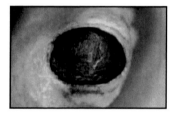

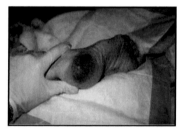

Figure 5.23. Stage I

Figure 5.24. Stage II

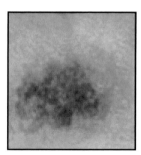

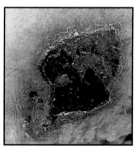

Figure 5.25. Stage III   **Figure 5.26.** Stage IV

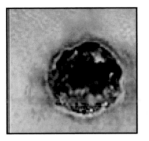   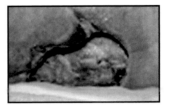

Figures 5.27.-5.30. illustrate steps in healing from Stage IV pressure ulcer to closure.

Figure 5.27. Hemostatisis (note bone)   **Figure 5.28.** Inflammation

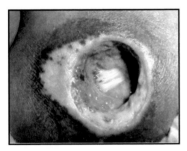   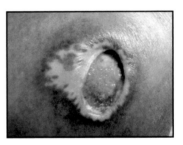

Figure 5.29. Proliferation   **Figure 5.30.** Remodeling

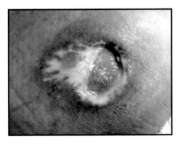   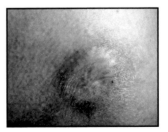

Figures 5.31.-5.33. Steps in Healing of Pressure Ulcer

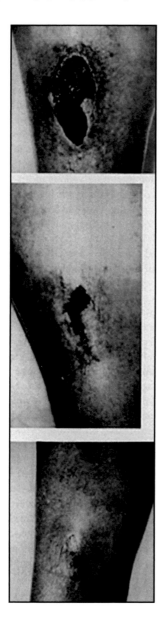

Figure 5.31. Inflammation, clean wound

Figure 5.32. Proliferation, wound edges are closing and wound is healing from inside out

Figure 5.33. Remodeling, scar tissue, fully healed

Hair

Hair is important to the appearance of men and women. Changes in hair may be due to a variety of reasons including nutrition. The hair is the only body structure that is completely renewable without scarring.

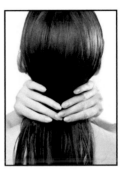

Hair has two separate structures; the follicle and the shaft. The follicle is in the skin and the shaft is the portion above the skin. It's normal to shed some hairs each day as old hairs are replaced by new ones. The follicular hair cycle is divided into three phases;

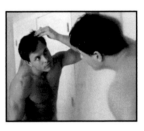

- Anagen
- Catagen
- Telogen

The anagen phase is the phase of active growth. The catagen phase marks follicular regression, and the telogen phase represents a resting period. In the human scalp, the anagen phase lasts approximately 3-4 years. Approximately 84% of scalp hairs are in the anagen phase. The catagen phase lasts approximately 2-3 weeks. Approximately 1-2% of scalp

Figure 5.34. Telogen Effluvium **Figure 5.35.** Anagen Effluvium

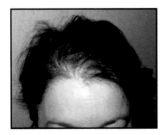
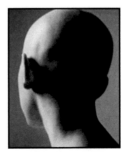

hairs are in the catagen phase. The telogen phase lasts approximately 3 months. About 10-15% of scalp hairs are in the telogen phase (Geiler, 2000; Rushton, 2002).

Practical Applications for NFPA: Alopecia

Alopecia or hair loss can happen for many reasons. Male-pattern baldness or androgenic alopecia is the most common cause of hair loss in men due to an inherited trait. Men who start losing their hair at an early age tend to develop more extensive baldness. In male-pattern baldness, hair loss typically results in a receding hair line and baldness on the top of the head. By age 35, about two-thirds of American men have some degree of appreciable hair loss and by age 50 approximately 85 % have significant hair thinning. A study using botulinum toxin A to treat androgenic alopecia has generated promising results (Freund, 2010). More research is needed to validate findings.

Female-pattern baldness causes hair to thin, but rarely leads to total baldness. The American Academy of Dermatology reports that 40 % of women have visible hair loss by age 40. Hormone changes during and after pregnancy trigger changes in the hair. Extreme stress from a major illness, very low calorie diets, rapid weight loss following bariatric surgery, underlying health problems, such as polycystic ovary syndrome or thyroid disease and certain medicines, can trigger hair loss about 2 months following the episode of illness. Patients may experience telogen effluvium or hair "coming out in handfuls." Hair loss following bariatric surgery has been associated with inadequate intakes of protein, iron, zinc and biotin (Aills, 2008; Kaidar-Person, 2008; Bruginsky, 2001; Geiler, 2000; Rushton, 2002; Jacques, 2006). More randomized studies are needed to determine optimal levels of supplementation.

Alopecia areata is an autoimmune disorder in which the immune system attacks the hair follicles. It may start as patchy hair loss and can progress to total hair loss. Some research on use of nutritional supplements has indicated that zinc and biotin supplementation may produce a beneficial effect (Jablonska, 1981; Ead, 1981; Camacho, 1999). More studies are needed to confirm these relationships.

Alopecia & Medications
Medications may increase hair loss by interfering with the normal cycle of scalp hair growth triggering telogen effluvium and anagen effluvium. Telogen effluvium is the most common form of drug-induced hair loss. It usually appears within two to four months after taking the drug. This condition causes the hair follicles to go into their resting phase (telogen) and fall out too early. Patients with telogen effluvium usually shed between 100 and 150 hairs a day. Refer to Figure 5.34.

Anagen effluvium is hair loss that occurs during the anagen phase of the hair cycle, when the hairs are actively growing. It prevents the matrix cells, which produce new hairs, from dividing normally. This type of hair loss usually occurs within a few days to weeks after taking the medication. It is a common side effect of some types of chemotherapy, causing loss of all of the hair on the head, eyebrows, eyelashes, and other body hairs. Refer to Figure 5.35.

Medications that list hair loss as a side effect include: chemotherapy, Coumadin (warfarin); Lopid (gemfibrozil); antidepressants; beta-blockers; non-steroidal anti-inflammatory drugs (NSAIDs); and drugs for gout, arthritis, birth control, and high blood pressure. Complete scalp hair loss is alopecia totalis. Hair loss from the entire body, including the eyebrows, eyelashes, and body hair, is alopecia universalis. Usually, hair grows back when the medication is discontinued, but some drugs may cause permanent hair loss, or trigger male or female pattern hair loss.

Hair Analysis

Some companies claim that they can assess nutritional status by analyzing hair clippings. They promise benefits such as identification of toxins and nutrient deficiencies which in turn cause imbalances in the body and illness. Some providers promise that their hair analysis will *'reveal which foods you should increase or eliminate for your unique metabolism'* and *'reveal the cause of poor health.'* Hair analysis is also promoted as a tool for detoxification. Hair analysis can detect some poisons such as arsenic and lead, but there are no testing standards presently. There is no evidence based research to support the use of hair analysis in assessing nutrition status. Hair analysis may be helpful in the future to assess trace minerals for which measurements of functional status are not well developed such as zinc, copper, chromium, and manganese. Hair can be used for deoxyribonucleic acid (DNA) testing and may be useful in the future as a noninvasive methodology to predict genetic predisposition to disease and effectiveness of medical nutrition therapy.

Clinical Nutrition Pearls: Hair

Hair loss may be due to medications, genetics, hormone shifts, stress of serious illness or surgery, and sub-optimal nutrient intake. Hair loss is an emotionally devastating experience for many patients and it may or may not grow back in its original condition, distribution and density. During the NFPA, note the appearance, texture and distribution of the hair. Review medical history and medications to determine possible contributors to alopecia. Evaluate nutrient density of the diet for protein, iron, zinc and biotin. Nutrition diagnoses that may apply include altered nutrition-related lab values, impaired nutrient utilization or suboptimal micro or macronutrient intake. Collaborate with healthcare team members on supplementation recommendations.

Nails

Human fingernails and toenails are complex structures involving six structures including the germinal matrix, ventral matrix, nail plate, eponychium, perionychium and hyponychium. Each of these structures has a specific function, and if disrupted can result in an abnormal appearing nail. Refer to Figure 5.36.

The germinal matrix or root is the portion of the nail beneath the skin and extends several millimeters into the finger or toe. It produces most of the volume of the nail and the nail bed. The nail plate is a keratinized structure that grows throughout life. The ventral matrix is the vascular bed that is responsible for nail growth and support. The underneath surface of the nail plate are grooves along the length of the nail that help anchor it to the nail bed. It lies protected between the lunula (white "half moon" at proximal edge of nail bed) and the hyponychium (junction between the free edge of the nail and the skin of the fingertip or toetip, that provides a waterproof barrier). The eponychium is the epidermal layer between the proximal nail fold and the dorsal aspect of the nail plate. The perioncyhium is the skin that overlies the nail plate on its sides. It is the site of hangnails, ingrown nails, and an infection of the skin called paronychia. (Williams, 2008).

The primary purpose of the nail is protection. Abnormalities of the nail are often caused by skin disease and infection

Figure 5.36. Nail Anatomy

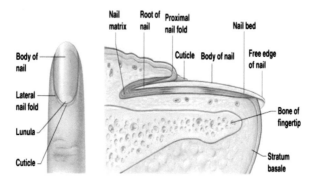

(most often fungal) but may also indicate general medical conditions including nutrient deficiencies.

Nail growth is continuous throughout the life cycle. Aging slows the rate of nail growth. In older adults, the distance between the free edge of the fingernail and the cuticle represents about 6 months compared with 3 months in children. Toenails grow at about 1/3 of the rate of fingernails. Timing of medical events can be estimated from the location of changes on the nail (Williams, 2008).

Practical Applications for NFPA: Nails & Nutrient Deficiencies

There are many nail abnormalities. Some are related to nutrient deficiencies. Other abnormalities are due to infections, diseases, trauma or side effects of medications. NFPA of fingernails must be done in adequate light. Evaluation includes the free edge, shape, color, paronychial tissue, lunula and growth rate. Observe the nail shape, surface color and presence of markings. Healthy nails (without polish) are typically pink.

Palpate the nail to assess texture and consistency. Healthy

nails are hard and immobile. Test for capillary refill in nail beds by pressing the nail tip or each side of the nail briefly and watch for a change in color. The nail appears blanched when squeezed. When pressure is released, the color returns to normal pink tones. The time it takes to return to original color is capillary refill time. Slower capillary refill times are common with respiratory and cardiovascular diseases that cause hypoxia and with dehydration (Murray, 2010). Bleeding around nails may indicate malnutrition. Nails that blanch poorly may suggest a deficiency of vitamins A or C. Flaky nail plates may suggest a magnesium deficiency (Cashman, 2010, Pogatshnik, 2011).

Koilonychia are spoon-shaped concave nails. This occurs normally in children and usually resolves with aging. To determine whether a nail is spooned, perform the water drop test. Place a drop of water on the nail. If the drop does not slide off, then the nail is flattened from early spooning. An experienced clinician can look at the nail and perform a "mental" water drop test. Causes of koilonychia include iron deficiency, malnutrition, protein deficiency especially indispensible amino acids methionine and cysteine, diabetes mellitus, systemic lupus and Raynaud's disease (Williams, 2008). Figure 5.37. illustrates koilonychia.

Brittle nails is a term used to describe soft, dry, weak or thin nails that split easily. Approximately 20 percent of the population has brittle nails. Thin brittle nails may suggest metabolic bone disease, thyroid disorder, magnesium deficiency or severe malnutrition (Williams, 2008). Brittle nails are illustrated in Figure 5.38.

There are many 'home remedies' for brittle nails that include foods and nutritional supplements including gelatin, biotin, calcium, zinc, magnesium, iron, and silicon. Gelatin is an incomplete protein that contributes little to total protein needs. There is no strong evidence that gelatin, calcium, biotin, zinc, magnesium or silicon supplementation improves brittle nails (Cashman, 2010;Derzavis, 1961; Hochman, 1993; Redi, 2000; Bauer, 1981; Sato, 1991, Scheinfeld, 2007;). Brittle nails have been reported in individuals with a vitamin A and selenium toxicity (Silverman , 1987; Bedwal 1993).

Beau's Lines or Transverse Linear Depressions are transverse line in the substance of the nail suggesting previous acute illness. The lines look as if a little furrow had been plowed across the nail. Illnesses producing Beau's Lines include severe infection, malnutrition, myocardial infarction, hypotension, hypocalcemia, uncontrolled diabetes, and surgery. Intermittent doses of immunosuppressive therapy or chemotherapy can also produce Beau's Lines. Severe zinc deficiency has also been proposed as a cause of Beau's Lines.

By noting its location on the nail, the approximate date of the illness associated with it can be determined. Also, the depth of the line provides a clue to the severity of the illness. Note Beau's Lines in Figure 5.39.-5.41. The two Beau's Lines suggest illnesses about 2 months apart (Williams, 2008).

Onychorrhexis is the presence of longitudinal striations or ridges. These ridges can simply be a sign of advanced age but it can also occur with rheumatoid arthritis or peripheral vascular disease. Central ridges can be caused by iron deficiency, folic acid deficiency, and malnutrition (Williams, 2008). Figure 5.42. illustrates a central ridge line. Central nail canal (median nail dystrophy) is associated with severe arterial disease, severe malnutrition and repetitive trauma (Williams, 2008). Refer to Figure 5.43.

Leukonychia are nails with nonuniform, white lines found in differing spots on one or more nails. They are thought to result from random minor trauma to the proximal nail bed and are of no medical significance. Refer to Figure 5.44.

Muehrcke's lines are pairs of transverse white lines that extend all the way across the nail, parallel to the edge of the lunula. The lines represent an abnormality of the vascular nail bed and disappear while the nail is depressed and blood is squeezed from the vessels beneath the nail. Muehrcke's lines occur in patients with hypoalbuminemia and disappear when the serum albumin level normalizes. They may be present in patients with nephrotic syndrome, liver disease, and malnutrition (Williams, 2008). Refer to Figure 5.45.

In patients with Terry's nails, most of the nail plate turns white with a dark band near the digital edge, and the lunula is obliterated. This condition is associated with severe liver disease, congestive heart failure, alcohol abuse and malnutrition. The condition is thought to be caused by a decrease in vascularity and an increase in connective tissue in the nail bed (Bickley, 2009). Refer to Figure 5.46.

In half-and-half nails the lunula is obliterated, the proximal nail turns white, and the distal nail turns brown. Increased melanin production may cause the distal part of the nail bed to turn brown. These nails can occur in patients with renal failure (Bickley, 2009). Refer to figure 5.47.

A change in the color of nails (independent of nail polish or other cosmetic treatments) may suggest a change in health status. White nails can be caused by anemia, edema or vascular condition, renal failure, cirrhosis, diabetes and chemotherapy. Refer to figure 5.48. Red or pink nails may be caused by malnutrition, lupus, carbon monoxide, angioma and polycythemia (Williams, 2008). Refer to Figure 5.49. Brown-gray nails may suggest vitamin B12 deficiency, diabetes mellitus or cardiovascular disease (Williams, 2008). Refer to Figure 5.50.

In yellow nail syndrome, nails thicken and new growth slows, resulting in discoloration. Nails affected with this condition may lack a cuticle and may detach from the nail bed in places. The lateral sides of the nail plate show exaggerated convexity, the lunula disappears, and the nail takes on a yellow hue. This syndrome has been reported in patients with pleural effusions, chronic bronchiectasis or sinusitis, internal malignancies, immunodeficiency syndromes, rheumatoid arthritis and lymphedema. The etiology of the change in nail hue may be related to impaired lymphatic drainage or to protein leakage from increased microvascular permeability. Refer to figure 5.51.

Nails with a bluish cast are the result of an increased concentration of deoxyhemoglobin (form of hemoglobin that circulates without oxygen) in cutaneous blood vessels. Blue nails are a sign of cyanosis. There are two forms of cyanosis. If the arterial blood oxygen level is low, cyanosis is central. Central cyanosis is best identified in the lips, oral mucosa and tongue. In dark skinned individuals, look at the palms, nails and soles of feet. If the arterial blood oxygen level is normal, cyanosis is peripheral. Peripheral cyanosis occurs when the cutaneous blood flow decreases or slows and tissues extract more oxygen than usual from the blood. It is a normal response to anxiety or a cold environment.

Nails with a blue cast may be a side effect of antimalarial medications (Bickley, 2009). Refer to Figure 5.52.

Digital clubbing is a term used to describe the bulbous uniform swelling of the soft tissue of the terminal phalanx of a digit with subsequent loss of the normal angle between the nail and the nail bed. There is normally a 160 degree angle between the nail base and the skin. Early clubbing is described as a 180 degree angle between the nail base and skin with spongy sensation. Late clubbing is described as greater than a 180 degree angle between the nail base and skin. Clubbing is usually bilateral and painless. It is a common clinical finding with cystic fibrosis, idiopathic pulmonary fibrosis, lung cancer, Hodgkin's lymphoma, cirrhosis of the liver, dysentery, Crohn's disease, ulcerative colitis and Graves' disease.

The nail feels soft and spongy when pressed toward the nail plate. The sponginess results from increased fibrovascular tissue between the nail and the phalanx. The terminal phalanx may appear large and bulging. The nail curves downward.

To assess for digital clubbing, ask patient to place the same finger from each hand with nail beds facing. In healthy nails, there is a diamond-shaped window, called Schamroth's window, between the two fingers when cuticle areas are placed next to each other. In clubbing, Schamroth's window is obliterated (Murray, 2010). Refer to Figures 5.53-5.55.

Clinical Nutrition Pearls: Nails
Patients rarely present with complaints related to the appearance of their nails. Many medical professionals are unfamiliar with common nail findings, especially those

associated with nutrient deficiencies. Nail abnormalities are usually medical diagnoses that may have concurrent nutrient deficiencies. Use NFPA to inspect nails as part of the nutrition assessment. Nutrition diagnoses that may apply include altered nutrition-related lab values, impaired nutrient utilization and suboptimal micro or macronutrient intakes. Collaborate with healthcare team members on supplementation recommendations. Changes in the color or appearance of the nail due to medications will persist during the course of the medication and until the nail grow out. Changes in the color or appearance of the nail due to chronic conditions will likely persist indefinitely.

Figure 5.37. Koilonychia   **Figure 5.38.** Brittle Nails

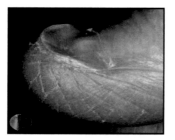 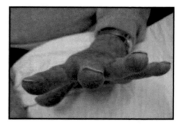

Figures 5.39.-5.41. Beau's Lines (note 2 lines on 5.39)

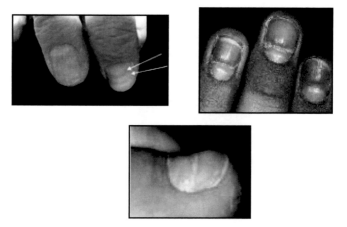

Figure 5.42. Onychorrhexis **Figure 5.43.** Central Nail Canal

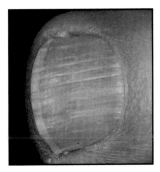
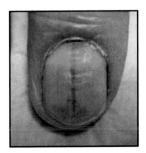

Figure 5.44. Leukonychia **Figure 5.45.** Muehrcke's Lines

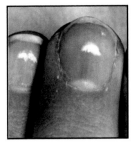
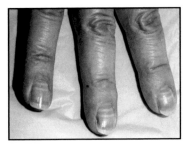

Figure 5.46. Terry's Nails **Figure 5.47.** Half-and-Half Nails

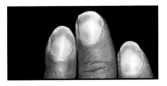
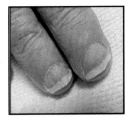

Figure 5.48. White Nails

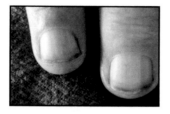

Figure 5.49. Red-pink Nails

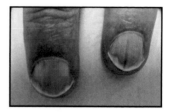

Figure 5.50. Brown-gray Nails

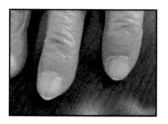

Figure 5.51. Yellow Nails

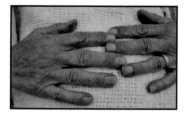

Figure 5.52. Blue Nails

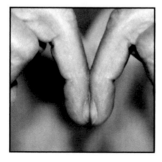

Figure 5.53. Clubbing

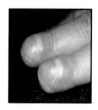

Figure 5.54. Schamroth's window

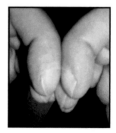

Figure 5.55. Clubbing

NFPA: Making Clinical Connections

References

Aills L, Blankenship J, Buffington C, et al. ASMBS allied health nutritional guidelines for the surgical weight loss patient. Surg Obes Relat Dis. 2008;4(Supp):73S–108S.

American Medical Directors Association (2007) Anemias in the long-term care setting. Clinical Practice Guideline. AMDA.

American Medical Directors Association (2008) Pressure ulcers in the long-term care setting. Clinical Practice Guideline. AMDA.

Bedwal, RS Selenium-its biological perspectives. Med Hypotheses, 1993:41:150-159.

Bickley,L. Bates guide to physical examination, 10th ed. Philadelphia,PA: Lippincott, 2009.

Braverman, IM (1986). Elastic fiber and microvascular abnormalities in aging skin. In: Gilchrest, BA ed. The aging skin, Dermatol Clin. 4:391.

Bruginsky A. Biotin supplementation as a treatment for alopecia post gastroplasty. Sao Paulo: Brazilian Institute of Homeopathic Studies. Specialization in Orthomolecular Nutrition and longevity. São Paulo, 2001:38

Camacho, FM. Zinc, aspartate, biotin and clobetasol propionate in the treatment of alopecia areata in childhood. Pediatr Dermatol 1999; 16:336.

Cashman, M. Nutrition and nail disease. Clin Dermatol, 2010 Jul-Aug;28(4):420-5.

Consortium for Spinal Cord Medicine, (2000). Pressure ulcer prevention and treatment following spinal cord injury: A clinical practice guideline for healthcare professionals. www.pva.org/NEWPVASITE/publications/cpg_pubs/PU.pdf.

Derzavis, JL The brittle nail: treatment and prevention with gelatin. Med Ann Dist Columbia, 1961: 30:133.

Ead, Rd. Oral zinc sulphate in alopecia areata- a double blind trial. Br J Dermatol, 1981:104: 483.

Ehrlich, HP & Hunt, TK (1968). Effects of cortisone and vitamin A on wound healing. Ann Surg 167:324.

Fawcett, RS, Linford,S Nail abnormalities: clues to systemic diseases. 2004 Am Fam Physician Mar 15;69(6) 1417-1424.

Freund BJ and Schwartz M. Treatment of male pattern baldness with botulinum toxin: A pilot study. Plast Reconstr Surg 2010 Nov; 126:246e.

Geiler CC. Metabolic disorders involving the hair. In: Camacho FM, , eds. Hair and its Disorders. Biology, Pathology and Management. London: Martin Dunitz; 2000:275–282.

Hochman, LG Brittle nails; response to daily biotin supplementation. Cutis 1993:51:303.

Horn, SD, Bender, SA, et al (2002). Description of the national pressure ulcer long-term care study. JAGS 50:1816-1825.

Horn, SD, Bender, SA, et al (2004). The National Pressure Ulcer Long-Term Care Study: Pressure Ulcer Development in Long-Term Care Residents. JAGS 52(3):359-367.

Jablonska, S zinc sulfate and alopecia totalis. Br J Dermatol, 1981:105: 485.

Jacques J. Micronutrition for the Weight Loss Surgery Patient. Edgemont, PA: Matrix Medical Communications; 2006:146–147.

Kaidar-Person, O., Person, B., Szomstein, S. et al. (2008) Nutritional deficiencies in morbidly obese patients: a new form of malnutrition? Part A: vitamins. Obesity Surgery, 18, 870–876. Epub 2008 March 4.

Kong, A, Acanthosis Nigricans: High Prevalence and Association with Diabetes in a Practice-based Research Network Consortium—A PRImary care Multi-Ethnic Network (PRIME Net) Study. J Am Board Fam Med. 2010;23(4):476-485.

Litchford, MD (2010). *Advanced Practitioner's Guide to Nutrition & Wound Healing.* Greensboro, NC: CASE Software & Books. www.casesoftware.com.

Litchford, MD (2011). *Laboratory Assessment of Nutritional Status: Bridging Theory & Practice.* Greensboro, NC: CASE Software & Books. www.casesoftware.com.

Litchford, MD (2009). *Common Denominators of Declining Nutritional Status.* Greensboro, NC: CASE Software & Books. www.casesoftware.com.

Lyder, CH, Preston, J, Grady, JN, et al (2001). Quality of care for hospitalized medicare patients at risk for pressure ulcers. Arch Intern Med 161:1549-1554.

Miller, J, Elston, D. Acanthosis Nigricans. http://emedicine.medscape.com/article/1102488-overview. Accessed September 2011.

Murray JF, Schraufnagel DE. History and physical examinations. In: Mason RJ, Broaddus VC, Martin TR, et al. Murray & Nadel's Textbook of Respiratory Medicine. 5th ed. Philadelphia, Pa: Saunders Elsevier;2010:chap 17.

National Pressure Ulcer Advisory Panel. Prevention and treatment of pressure ulcers. Washington DC: NPUAP; 2010.

Otto DE, Wang X, Tijerina SL, Reyna ME, Farooqi MI. A Comparison of Blood Pressure, Body Mass Index, and Acanthosis Nigricans in School-Age Children. J Sch Nurs. Mar 24 2010

Pogatshnik, C Nutrition focused physical examination: skin, nails, hair, eyes and oral cavity. DNS Support Line 2011, 33(2), 7-13.

Potts, JF (1990). Sunlight, sunburn and sunscreens. Postgrad Med. 87:52.

Redi, IF Calcium supplementation and nail quality. NJM 2000: 343: 1817.

Rushton DH. Nutritional factors and hair loss. Clin Exp Dermatol 2002;27:396–404.

Sato, S. Iron deficiency: structural and microchemical changes in hair, nails and skin. Semin Dermatol, 1991:10: 313-318.

Scheinfeld, N. Vitamins and minerals: their role in nail health and disease. J Drugs Dermatol, 2007 Aug;6(8):782-7.

Schwartz, RA. Carotenemia. Medscape eMedicine, 5/27/2011. http://emedicine.medscape.com/article/1104368-overview. accessed 9/2011.

Selvaag, E, Bohmer, T(2002). Reduced serum concentrations of riboflavin & ascorbic acid, and blood thiamine pyrophosphate & pyridoxal-5-phosphate in geriatric patients with & without pressure ulcers, J Nutr Health Aging. 6(1):75-77.

Silverman, AK Hypervitaminosis A syndrome. J am Dermatol 1987:16:1027-1039.

Williams, W Examining the fingernails when evaluating presenting symptoms in elderly patients.2008. Medscape Family Medicine. http://www.medscape.org/viewarticle/571916

Chapter 6
Tools for Assessing Hydration Status

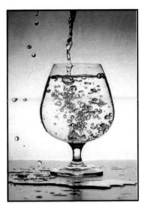

Water is one of the six main categories of essential nutrients. It is often ignored by healthcare providers as evidenced by the accuracy rate of clinical diagnoses for dehydration and hypovolemia by physicians and nurses (Bennett, 2004; Thomas, 2004). Yet water is essential for survival.
Total body water compromises 50-60% of the weight of adults. About 2/3 of the total body water is present in the intracellular fluid and 1/3 is extracellular fluid. Under normal circumstances, the movement of water between water compartments occurs by the actions of osmosis and hydrostatic pressure. Changes in hydration status may be insidious or remarkable.

Formulae commonly used to estimate water requirements are based on consensus rather than evidence based guidelines (IOM, 2005). In the MDS 3.0, Section J, the presence of dehydration is defined as the presence of two or more potential indicators. Indicators are divided into three categories: insufficient fluid intake, clinical signs of dehydration, and increased fluid losses. The Resident assessment Instrument (RAI) Manual states that the recommended intake level for fluid has changed from 2,500 mL to 1,500 mL per day to reflect current practice standards, however, individualized assessments may estimate higher water needs (CMS, 2011).

Some questions to consider in assessing for dehydration or hypovolemia include:
• Has water intake changed due to a change in medical condition or a change in medications?
• Is the patient having increased difficulty swallowing medications?
• Is the patient refusing medications more frequently?
• Is the patient dependent on others to access water or for other reasons?
• Is the patient more difficult to understand (i.e. very soft voice or garbled speech)?
• Is the patient more confused or combative?
• Does the patient self-impose water restrictions due to unscientific beliefs?
• Does the patient have more difficulty with water than thicker beverages (i.e. tomato juice, milk shake)?
• Look at the patient's face. Do the eyes have a sunken appearance?
• Do the skin, lips, tongue and mucous membranes appear dry?

Practical Applications for NFPA: Dehydration

Dysregulation of water balance includes dehydration, hypovolemia and overhydration. Each condition can be life-threatening in infants and older adults. There is not one single lab test or clear cut diagnostic criteria that delineate dysregulation of water balance. Dehydration, hypovolemia and overhydration are medical diagnoses.

Dehydration has been described by serum sodium values as hypertonic or hypernatremic dehydration, hypotonic or hyponatremic dehydration and isotonic or isonatremic dehydration (Ellsbury, 2003). However Thomas (2004) differentiated dehydration from hypovolemia. Dehydration was defined as water loss that exceeds sodium loss resulting in hypernatremia and hyperosmolality. The diagnostic criteria include serum sodium > 145 mmol/L and serum osmolality of > 300 mmol/kg H20. Hypovolemia was defined as loss of water from both intravascular and extravascular fluid compartments resulting in decreased tissue perfusion. The diagnostic criteria include serum osmolality of > 295 mmol/kg H20 and BUN/creatinine ratio > 20. Hypovolemia is also referred to as hypotonic hypovolemic hyponatremia.

Diagnosis requires a global, interdisciplinary assessment and analysis of many factors including estimated daily water intake. Overhydration is also discussed in Chapter 4.

NFPA for water dysregulation begins with a review of the medical record for signs and conditions noted in table 6.1. Physical signs of dehydration are less specific in the elderly than in younger adults. Medications and mouth breathing are two confounding factors that contribute to dry mucous membranes and xerostomia. Chronic xerostomia may result in difficulty swallowing medications and food. It may exacerbate a pre-existing dysphagia resulting in reduced food and water intake. Xerostomia may affect the ability to speak or to speak clearly. Review the food and water intake records for patterns of reduced water intake and observe at mealtime.

 NFPA for dehydration and hypovolemia require inspection and palpation. Physical signs of dehydration include dry, scaling skin with cracked lips, cheilosis, dry mucous membranes specifically around the eyes, lips, mouth and tongue. The tongue may appear sunken and have deep dry furrows. Look at the corners of the mouth for signs of splitting or sores. The eyes may have a sunken appearance

due to dehydration or atrophy of facial muscles or loss
of orbital fat due to malnutrition. Degrees of severity of
dehydration associated with specific clinical findings are
noted on Table 6.2.

Table 6.1. Medical Conditions Associated with Increased Risk of
Dehydration

Signs	Conditions & Contributing Factors
Abnormal lab test results	Elderly
Constipation	Low BMI
Diarrhea	Impaired thirst response
Disorientation	High protein diet
Dry mucous membranes	History of dysphagia
Dry sunken tongue, furrows	Compromised cognitive status
Fever	Dependent eaters
Hypotension	Depression
Increased fluid losses	Infection
Increased respiratory rate	Chronic co-morbidities (stroke, diabetes, CHF)
Excessive urination	Skin breakdown
Low urinary output or dark urine	Draining wounds
Perfuse diaphoresis	Unplanned weight loss
Poor skin turgor	Meds that promote fluid loss
Sunken eyes	NPO or fluid restriction
Tachycardia	Prior hospitalization for dysregulation of water balance
Vertigo on sitting/standing	Very hot environment
Thready or faint pulse	
Vomiting	

Check the turgor or elasticity of the skin for tenting. Lightly
pinch the skin using the thumb and forefinger. In well-
hydrated adults, the skin will return to the normal contour

within 3 seconds. If the skin remains elevated or tented for more than 3 seconds, the turgor is decreased. The relative speed with which the skin resumes its normal appearance after stretching or compression is an indicator of skin hydration. Turgor is slower in older adults and is not a reliable indicator of dehydration. Do not check skin turgor on patients with extremely thin skin or who bruise easily. Preferred sites to evaluate for tenting are the sternum and on the inner aspect of the thigh. Many clinicians use the top of the hand where skin tends to be loose in older adults.

Table 6.2. Clinical Findings for Degrees of Dehydration

Signs	Mild	Moderate	Severe
Level of Consciousness	Alert	Lethargic	Unresponsive
Capillary Refill	2 Seconds	4 Seconds	> 4 Seconds, Cool Limbs
Mucous Membranes	Normal	Dry	Parched or Cracked
Tears	Normal	Decreased	Absent
Heart Rate	Slight Increase	Increased	Rapid
Respiratory Rate	Normal	Increased	Hyperpnea
Blood Pressure	Normal	Normal, but Orthostasis	Decreased
Pulse	Normal	Thready	Faint
Skin turgor	Normal	Slow	Tenting
Fontanel	Normal	Depressed	Sunken
Eyes	Normal	Sunken	Very Sunken
Urine Output	Decreased	Oliguria	Oliguria or Anuria
Urine color	Normal	Light yellow	Dark yellow

Check capillary refill time. First, palpate nails to assess the circulation, then gently squeeze each nail between thumb

and index finger. The nail appears
blanched (white) when squeezed.
The color should return to normal
pink tones within < 2-3 seconds.
The time it takes to return to
original color is capillary refill time.
Interpretation of capillary refill time
is noted on Table 6.2.

Figure 6.1 Capillary Refill

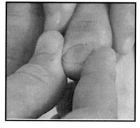

Figure 6.2 Urine Colors

Check the color of the urine either visually or
review the nurses notes for data. A clear
light straw color suggests that water needs
are being met. Darker urine (golden or
brown) may suggest insufficient water
intake. Some medications and micronutrients change the normal color of urine.
Refer to Figure 6.2.

Once physical signs of dehydration or
hypovolemia are suspected or observed, look
for corroborating evidence in the medical record and food
and water intake data. Evaluate changes in weight. Rapid
weight loss is often due to loss of body water. Review lab
test results for serum sodium, BUN, albumin, hemoglobin,
hematocrit, osmolality, glucose and other tests to identify
a pattern of findings. Compare current lab test results with
historic data. Individuals who are normally hyponatremic
may have normal sodium values when in fact the finding is
elevated compared to baseline (Litchford, 2011).

Using the food and water intake data, estimate the average
daily water intake and compare to estimated water
requirements. Consider estimating preformed water in food

and metabolic water production. Food contributes about 20-25% of the water requirement and metabolic water production contributes about 9-10% of water requirement (IOM, 2005).

If severe dehydration is suspected, calculate water deficit to determine water depletion. Water deficits can be estimated using serum sodium and usual body weight (kg). The formula is based on the assumption that water contributes about 50% of total body weight in adults. It also assumes that the average extracellular concentration of sodium is 140 mEq/L. See Table 6.3 (AMDA, 2001).

Table 6.3. Equation to Estimate Water Deficit

Estimated water deficit = $$\frac{[\text{serum Na} \times \text{body wt(kg)} \times 0.5]}{140} - [\text{body wt(kg)} \times 0.5]$$
Example: Wt today 50 kg, Na 154 mmol/L $$\frac{[154 \times 50(\text{kg}) \times 0.5]}{140} - [50(\text{kg}) \times 0.5] =$$ 27.5L – 25 L = ~ 2.5 L water deficit

Other Clinical Practice Guidelines: Dehydration

Compare your findings to other clinical practice guidelines. The American Medical Directors Association (AMDA) Clinical Practice Guideline for diagnosis of dehydration uses these criteria:

- Suspicion of low intake or excessive output
- 2 or more physiological or functional signs or symptoms suggesting dehydration
  - BUN: Creatinine ratio > 25:1 OR
  - Orthostasis OR
  - Pulse > 100 beats/minute OR
  - Change in pulse of 10-20 beats/minute > baseline with a change in position (AMDA, 2001)

Practical Applications for NFPA: Overhydration

Overhydration occurs when there is an increase in the extracellular fluid volume. The fluid shifts from the extracellular compartment to the interstitial fluid compartment which can lead to a decreased sodium concentration in the blood (Chernoff, 1994; IOM, 2005; Whitmire, 2008). Common causes of overhydration are noted on Table 6.4

Table 6.4. Common Causes of Overhydration

Increased capillary hydrostatic pressure (CHF)
Decreased colloid osmotic pressure (hypoalbuminemia)
Lymphatic obstruction (following surgery)
Organ failure (kidney or liver)
Decreased physical activity

Symptoms of overhydration and hyponatremia include shortness of breath, orthopnea, edema, increased blood pressure, tachycardia, distended neck veins, and ultimately death if left untreated (Chernoff, 1994a; Schrier, 2006; Whitmire, 2008). Fluid accumulation may be insidious or remarkable. Some questions to consider in assessing for overhydration:

• Has water intake changed due to change in medical condition or a change in medications?
• Is the patient having increased difficulty breathing?
• Is the patient short of breath at meals or talking?
• Are there signs of wheezing?
• Is the patient asking for water or other beverages more frequently?
• Has the patient gained weight rapidly without an increase in food intake?
• Is there evidence of reduced food intake due to fatigue?

NFPA for overhydration includes inspection and palpation. The advanced level practitioner may be trained to assess for pulmonary edema, ascites and pleural edema using percussion and auscultation.

Begin NFPA by reviewing the medical record for rapid, unplanned weight gain, abnormal lab test results, and nursing notes specific to abdominal distention, dyspnea, wheezing, 'crackles' or 'rales.' Crackles or rales are abnormal breath sounds usually caused by excessive fluid within the airways. The fluid could be due to an exudate, as in pneumonia or other infections of the lung, or a transudate in congestive heart failure. Inspect and palpate extremities for edema. Observe the jugular neck vein for distention while patient is lying at a 45 degree angle. Stoop down to look at eye level. Collaborate with other medical team members on abnormal findings. See Figure 6.10.

Figures 6.3-6.8. are examples of physical signs of dehydration and hypovolemia.

Figure 6.3. Tenting of Skin   **Figure 6.4.** Dry Tongue

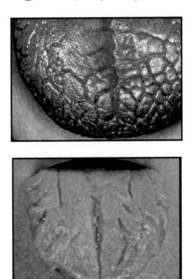

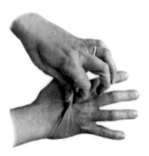

Figure 6.5. Dry Tongue (Note furrows in tongue)

Figure 6.6. Normal Lips vs. Chapped Lips

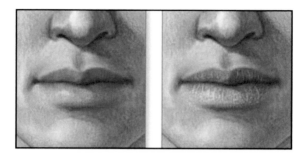

Figure 6.7. Cheilitis   **Figure 6.8.** Cheilosis

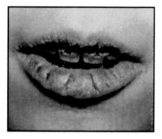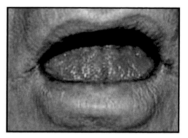

Figures 6.9-6.10. are examples of physical signs of overhydration.

Figure 6.9. Pitting Edema   **Figure 6.10.** Distended Neck Vein

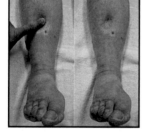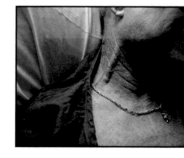

Clinical Nutrition Pearls: Hydration

Diseases and disorders associated with water dysregulation are medical diagnoses. Inappropriate intervention strategies can create additional problems for the patient with declining nutrition status. Dehydration is the most common fluid electrolyte disorder of frail older adults living in community or institutional settings (Lavizzo-Mourey, 1988). Mortality of patients/residents with dehydration is high if not treated adequately and in some studies exceeds 50% (Bourdel-Marchesson, 2004: Warren, 1996; Mahowald, 1981). In terms of morbidity, several studies have shown an association between severe dehydration and poor mental function (Seymour, 1980; Wilson, 2003). Other studies found that dehydration was a significant risk factor for developing thromboembolic complications, infectious disease, kidney stones and obstipation (fecal impaction) (Embon, 1990; Wrenn, 1989).

Nutrition diagnoses associated with dehydration and hypovolemia may include suboptimal fluid intake, swallowing difficulties, altered GI function, impaired nutrient utilization, and unintentional weight loss. Monitor the effectiveness of nutrition interventions closely because as water deficits increase in severity so do the signs and symptoms of dehydration.

Overhydration often masks other problems including abnormal laboratory values and weight loss. Considerable fluid buildup in the lungs and peritoneal cavity is a significant change requiring further assessment to determine the root cause. Note that overhydration is a medical diagnosis and requires a multidisciplinary approach to ensure that care needs are met. The nutrition professional is identifying nutrition diagnoses that may be contributing to overhydration. Nutrition diagnoses associated with overhydration may include excessive fluid intake, excessive sodium intake, malnutrition, unintentional weight gain, disordered eating pattern, and undesirable food choices. Monitor the effectiveness of nutrition interventions closely because changes in hydration status can shift quickly.

References

American Dietetic Association Evidence Analysis Library. What is the best clinical and/or biochemical parameter for hydration status in the adult (19-64 years)? http://www.adaevidencelibrary.com/conclusion.cfm?conclusion_statement_id=250805 Published 2007. Accessed November 1, 2011.

American Medical Directors Association (2001). Dehydration and fluid maintenance. Columbia, MD: ADMA.

Bennett JA, (2004) Unrecognized chronic dehydration in older adults: examining prevalence rate and risk factors. J Gerontol Nurs, 11:22-8.

Bickley,L. Bates guide to physical examination, 10th ed. Philadelphia,PA: Lippincott, 2009.

Bourdel-Marchasson I, Proux S, Dehail P, (2004) One-year incidence of hyperosmolar states and prognosis in a geriatric acute care unit. Gerontology;50:171-6.

Centers for Medicare and Medicaid Services (CMS): MDS 3.0 for Nursing Home. http://www.cms.gov/NursingHomeQuality-Inits/30_NHQIMDS30TechnicalInformation.asp#Top OfPage.htm. Accessed November 17, 2011.

CMS: State Operations Manual, Appendix PP-Guidance to Surveyors for Long Term Care Facilities. Section 483.20(b) Utilization Guidelines for Completion of the RAI. http://cms.hhs.gov/manuals/Downloads/som107ap_pp_guidelines_ltcf.pdf. Accessed November 17, 2011.

Chernoff R. Nutritional requirements and physiological changes in aging. Nutr Rev. 1994;52(8)(suppl):S3-S5.

Embon OM, Rose GA, Rosenbaum T. (1990)Chronic dehydration stone disease. Br J Urol ;66:357-62.

Faes, MC, Spigt, MG, Rikkert, MG (2007) Dehydration in geriatrics.Geriatrics & Aging 10(9):590-596

Grandjean AC, Campbell SM. Hydration: Fluids for life. A monograph by the North American Branch of the International Life Science Institute. Washington DC: ILSA North America; 2004.

Institute of Medicine. Dietary Reference Intakes for water, potassium, sodium, chloride & sulfate. Washington, DC: NAS, 2005.

Jequier E, Constant F. Water as an essential nutrient: The physiological basis of hydration. Eur J Clin Nutr. 2010;64:115-123.

Kant AK, Graubard BI, Atchison EA. Intakes of plain water, moisture in foods and beverages, and total water in the adult US population—nutritional, meal pattern, and body weight correlates: National Health and Nutrition Examination Surveys 1999–2006. Am J Clin Nutr. 2009;90:655-663.

Lavizzo-Mourey R (1988) Risk factors for dehydration among elderly nursing home residents. JAGS;36:213-8.

Litchford, MD, Laboratory Assessment of Nutritional Status: Bridging Theory & Practice. 2011. Greensboro, NC: CASE Software & Books. www.casesoftware.com

Mahowald JM.(1981) Hypernatremia in the elderly: relation to infection and mortality. JAGS ;29:177-80.

Manz F, Johner SA, Wentz A, Boeing H, Remer T. Water balance throughout the adult life span in a German population. Br J Nutr. 2011;16:1-9.

Noakes TD, Wilson G. Peak rates of diuresis in healthy humans during oral fluid overload. S Afr Med J. 2001;91:852-857.

Popkin BM, D'Anci KE, Rosenberg IH. Water, hydration, and health. Nutr Rev. 2010;68(8):439-458.

Raman A, Schoeller DA, Subar AF, et al. Water turnover in 458 American adults 40-79 year of age. Am J Physiol Renal Physiol. 2004;286:F394-F401.

Schrier RW. Body water homeostasis: Clinical disorders of urinary dilution and concentration. J Am Soc Nephrol. 2006;17:1820-1832.

Schwartz, R Carotenemia. e-Medicine Medscape. May, 2011. http://emedicine.medscape.com/article/1104368-overview

Seymour DG, Henschke PJ, (1980). Acute confusional states and dementia in the elderly: the role of dehydration/volume depletion, physical illness and age. Age Ageing 1980;9:137-46.

Thomas DR, Cote TR, Lawhorne L. Understanding clinical dehydration and its treatment. J Am Med Dir Assoc. 2008;9:292-301.

Thomas DR, Tariq SH, Makhdomm S, Haddad R, Moinuddin A. Physician misdiagnosis of dehydration in older adults. J Am Med Dir Assoc. 2004;5(suppl):S31-S34.

Warren JL, Harris T, Phillips C(1996) Dehydration in older adults. JAMA; 275:911-2.

Weinberg, AD & Minaker, KL (1995) Dehydration: evaluation and management in older adults. JAMA, 274: 1552-1556.

Whitmire SJ. Nutrition-focused evaluation and management of dysnatremias. Nutr Clin Pract. 2008;23:108-121.

Wilson M, Morley J (2003). Impaired cognitive function and mental performance in mild dehydration. Eur J Clin Nutr. 57:S24-9.

Wrenn K.(1989) Fecal impaction. NEJM 321:658-62.

Chapter 7
Digestive System

Figure 7.1. Oral Cavity

NFPA of the digestive system includes the path food travels from the mouth to the rectum. Examination techniques include inspection, palpation, and auscultation. This chapter includes a range of assessment techniques. The patient's medical history and alterations in nutrition status will

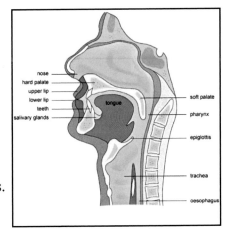

determine the components of NFPA to incorporate into the assessment. Remember that this is a focused assessment. Additional training may be required to learn the techniques of doing an oral assessment and interpretation of bowel sounds.

Figure 7.2. Bone of Skull

Oral Cavity

The oral cavity is defined as the space between the lips and pharynx. Muscles involved in chewing are all innervated by the trigeminal nerve.

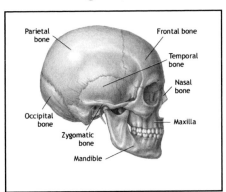

Muscles used for mastication include the temporalis which elevates, retracts, and assists in closing the mandible, the masseter which elevates and closes the mandible, the medial which also elevates the mandible and aids in its closure, the lateral pterygoid which depresses, opens, and protrudes the mandible, as well as moving it laterally.

Changes in to the oral cavity due to disease, injury, medications, damage to the cranial nerves and wasting of the muscles involved in chewing and swallowing can increase the risk of aspiration and result in dysphagia.

Figure 7.3. Muscles for Mastication: Temporalis & Masseter

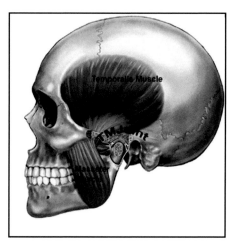

Some questions to consider as part of the oral assessment:
• Have your eating patterns changed over the last week or months?
• Has the amount of food eaten changed?
• How does your typical food intake for a day this week compare to 6 or 12 months ago?
• Are there certain foods that you no longer eat? If yes, why?
• Do any foods cause heartburn or belching?
• Does your mouth feel dry?
• Are you experiencing any nausea or vomiting?

- Do you have increased difficulty swallowing medications?
- Do you have any pain with chewing or swallowing?
- Do you have any sores or lumps inside your mouth?
- Do you hear the dentures 'click' while the patient speaks?
- When was the last time you saw the dentist for a check-up? Did you follow the dentist's recommendations?

Practical Applications for NFPA: Oral Cavity

During the general survey observe the face, lips and mouth for cheilosis, xerostomia, swollen parotid glands, and stomatitis. Next, ask the patient if you may look inside his/her mouth and explain that you would like to do a global assessment of their tongue, mouth and teeth. Be sure to follow the standard and universal precautions to protect the patient and yourself from the spread of infectious diseases. Tools needed to complete an oral exam include gloves, tongue depressor and light source that is adequate to visualize the back of the mouth. Refer to Figure 7.4.

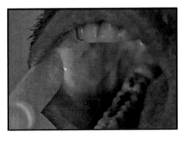

Figure 7.4. Oral Exam

First, ask the patient to stick out his/her tongue. Inspect the tongue for signs of dehydration and atrophy of papillae. Using a tongue depressor and light source, visually observe and feel all oral surfaces including lips, gums, tongue, palate, mouth floor, and cheek lining. Check for oral cleanliness, abnormal mouth tissue, abnormal teeth, and inflamed or bleeding gums. Using a gloved hand, palpate the oral mucosa for masses, check for loose teeth, and loose fitting dentures. Note food debris if present. Observe for signs of discomfort. Discard the tongue depressor and gloves after use.

Decide how to document your findings. One option is to classify the findings as healthy, early signs of problems and unhealthy. Refer to Figures 7.5-7.18. NFPA does not replace a dental evaluation. Collaborate with the medical team for areas of early or evident signs of dental problems.

Oral Assessment in Long Term Care Settings

In a long term care setting, there are specific requirements for completing the oral assessment. Oral health is a key component of health related quality of life for older adults because it impacts overall well being and nutrition status. The oral assessment was added to MDS 3.0 because assessing dental status can help identify residents who may be at risk for aspiration, malnutrition, pneumonia, endocarditis and poorly controlled of diabetes. Nutrition professionals working in CMS certified nursing facilities may be asked to do the oral assessment and to complete Section L of MDS 3.0. The RAI manual outlines the steps for the oral assessment and characteristics to document on the MDS 3.0. To complete Section L, the assessor must inspect and palpate the oral cavity for 6 characteristics noted on Table 7.1. Supplementary training materials are available at www.cms.gov.

Table 7.1. Oral Assessment, MDS 3.0, Section L

A. Broken or loosely fitting full or partial denture (chipped, cracked, uncleanable or loose)
B. No natural teeth or tooth fragment(s) (edentulous)
C. Abnormal mouth tissue (ulcers, masses, oral lesions, including denture or partial if one is worn)
D. Obvious or likely cavity or broken natural teeth
E. Inflamed or bleeding gums or loose natural teeth
F. Mouth or facial pain, discomfort or difficulty with chewing
G. Unable to examine
Z. None of the above

Start the assessment reviewing the dental history and other data pertinent in the medical record. Observe the resident at one or more meals to determine if chewing problems or mouth pain are evident. Plan a time to complete the 'hands on' portion of the assessment. A nursing assistant or other healthcare professional may need to be present for emotional support of the resident.

Begin the 'hands on' assessment by asking questions about difficulties eating. During the interview, listen for 'clicking' dentures. Dentures become loose because the mouth naturally changes with age. Bone and gum ridges can recede or shrink, causing jaws to align differently and can cause dentures to fit less securely. Significant weight loss can also affect the fit of dentures. Loose dentures can cause health problems, including sores and infections. A loose denture also makes chewing more difficult and may contribute to unplanned weight loss. Some questions to consider include:
• Are you having any difficulty chewing cooked or raw foods?
• Do you have mouth or facial pain when chewing?
• Do you have any broken teeth or teeth that feel rough to your tongue?
• Do your gums bleed easily?
• When was the last time you saw your dentist?
• Did you follow the recommendations of your dentist?
• Do you have any lumps or masses in your mouth?
• Do you wear dentures or partials? If yes ask, how long have you had the dentures or partials?
• If resident or family/significant other reports that the resident recently had dentures or partials, but they do not have them at the facility, ask for a reason.
• If resident or family/significant other reports that the resident has dentures or partials, but they do not wear

them at meal time, ask for a reason.
• Please remove the dentures or partials so that I can examine them for chips or cracks.

Next, ask the patient if you may look inside his/her mouth and explain that you would like to do a global assessment of their tongue, mouth and teeth. Ask residents who wear dentures or partials to remove these as part of the assessment. Some residents have dentures or partials, but do not wear them for meals.

Be sure to follow the standard and universal precautions to protect the patient and yourself from the spread of infectious diseases. Tools needed to complete an oral exam include gloves, tongue depressor and light source that is adequate to visualize the back of the mouth. Visually observe and feel all oral surfaces including lips, gums, tongue, palate, mouth floor, and cheek lining. Check for abnormal mouth tissue, abnormal teeth, or inflamed or bleeding gums. The assessor should use his or her gloved fingers to adequately feel for masses or loose teeth. Also note any food debris. Collaborate with the interdisciplinary team on abnormal findings. Discard the tongue depressor and gloves after use.

The oral assessment does not replace routine dental evaluations by a dentist. The Omnibus Reconciliation Act (OBRA) Guidelines allow all residents to refuse medical assessments, care and treatments. Residents who refuse the oral assessment, are uncooperative or who have areas of concern in the oral cavity should be referred for a dental evaluation. A change in diet consistency may be appropriate. RDNs may be required to complete the nursing home mandated training on doing an oral assessment and on standard and universal precautions. Refer to Figures 7.5-7.18 for examples of early and advanced signs of oral health problems.

Figures 7.5.-7.6. Lips: Signs of Trouble, Unhealthy

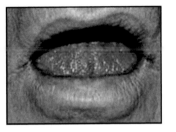 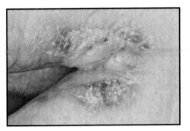

Figures 7.7.-7.8. Tongue: Signs of Trouble, Unhealthy

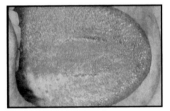 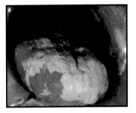

Figures 7.9.-7.10. Gums: Signs of Trouble, Unhealthy

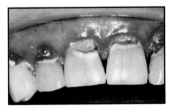 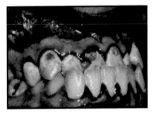

Figures 7.11.-7.12. Teeth: Signs of Trouble, Unhealthy

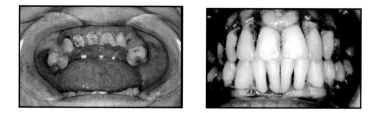

Figures 7.13.-7.14. Oral Hygiene: Signs of Trouble, Unhealthy

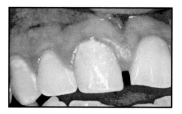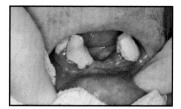

Figures 7.15.-7.16. Dentures: Signs of Trouble, Unhealthy

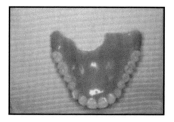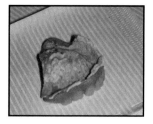

Figure 7.17. Mouth Ulcer   **Figure 7.18.** Stomatitis

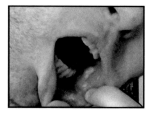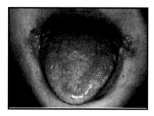

Cranial Nerves

The cranial nerves are composed of twelve pairs of nerves that emanate from the nervous tissue of the brain through openings in the skull to target tissues. Sensory components transmit nerve impulses from sensory organs to the brain. Table 7.2. lists the cranial nerves and their functions. The olfactory nerve, trigeminal nerve, facial nerve, glossopharyngeal nerve, vagus nerve, spinal accessory and hypoglossal nerve are involved in the process of eating. NFPA will include assessment of the olfactory nerve, trigeminal nerve, glossopharyngeal nerve, vagus nerve, and hypoglossal nerve.

Practical Applications for NFPA: Olfactory Nerve Assessment (Cranial Nerve I)

The olfactory nerve is located in the olfactory mucosa of the upper parts of the nasal cavity. During breathing air molecules attach to the olfactory mucosa and stimulate the olfactory receptors of cranial nerve I and electrical activity is transduced into the olfactory bulb. Olfactory bulb cells then transmit electrical activity to other parts of the central nervous system via the olfactory tract.

Unplanned weight loss, anorexia and a reduced sense of smell may be related to an altered olfactory nerve function. Patients often notice changes in their sense of smell and appetite before the clinician identifies a problem. Some questions to consider include:
• Do you think you have a reduced sense of smell?
• Do notice the aroma of foods, flowers or perfume?
• Have you had unplanned weight loss in the last 6-12 months?

To test for olfactory nerve function, prepare two unmarked

containers of aromatic products such as coffee, cinnamon or vanilla extract. Tell the patient you are going to test their sense of smell. Ask the patient close his/her eyes. Occlude one nostril and place the aromatic product under the open nostril. Ask the patient to identify the aroma. Test each nostril with one or two different substances. Allow ample time between aromas to prevent smell fatigue. Refer to Figure 7.19.

Table 7.2. Major Functions of Cranial Nerves

Cranial Nerve:	Major Functions:
I Olfactory	sense of smell
II Optic	vision
III Oculomotor	eyelid and eyeball movement
IV Trochlear	eyeball movement
V Trigeminal	chewing face & mouth touch & pain
VI Abducens	eyeball movement
VII Facial	controls most facial expression secretion of tears & saliva taste
VIII Vestibulocochlear (auditory)	hearing equilibrium sensation
IX Glossopharyngeal	tongue & taste throat senses carotid blood pressure
X Vagus	senses aortic blood pressure slows heart rate stimulates digestive organs' taste pharyngeal (gag) reflex
XI Spinal Accessory	controls head, neck and shoulder movement controls swallowing
XII Hypoglossal	controls tongue movements speech, chewing & swallowing

Trigeminal Nerve Assessment (Cranial Nerve V)

The trigeminal nerve is the largest of the cranial nerves and is composed of three branches. One of the sensory branches is distributed to the muscles of mastication, (i.e. temporalis and masseter muscles) face, oral cavity, pharynx and tongue.

To assess the motor function, ask the patient to the clench the jaw. Note the strength of the muscles and contractions controlled by the temporalis and masseter muscles. All muscles, including those used for chewing will atrophy with aging, unplanned weight loss, malnutrition and lack of use. Refer to Chapter 4 for more information on wasting of temporalis muscle. Refer to Figure 7.20.

Glossopharyngeal & Vagus Nerve Assessment (Cranial Nerves IX & X)

The glossopharyngeal nerve is related to the tongue and the pharynx. The vagus nerve is the longest of the cranial nerves, traveling from the brain stem through organs in the neck, thorax and abdomen. These nerves carry gustatory information to the brain.

Symptoms of damage to the vagus nerve depend on the severity of the nerve damage, the location of the injury and whether nearby blood vessels are also affected. The primary concerns for NFPA include altered speaking and a lost gag or pharyngeal reflex resulting in increased risk for aspiration, choking and dysphagia. Damage to the vagus nerve can result in trouble with moving the tongue while speaking, or hoarseness of the voice if the branch leading to the larynx is damaged. Also, the vagus nerve controls many muscles in the palate and tongue which, if damaged, can cause dysphagia. The gag or pharyngeal reflex is controlled by the vagus nerve, and damage may cause this reflex to be lost, increasing the risk of choking on saliva or food.

Unplanned weight loss, avoiding thin liquids, a reduced dietary intake, and signs of dehydration may be related to an altered glossopharyngeal and vagus nerve function. Patients may not notice changes in their ability to speak clearly or difficulty swallowing foods and beverages before the clinician identifies a problem. Mealtime observation is vital. Some questions to consider include :
• Do you have increased difficulty swallowing water compared to other beverages?
• Do foods or beverages 'go down the wrong way' at meals? If yes, ask how often?
• Do you have any pain with swallowing?
• Do some foods 'stick' in your throat?

Tools needed to test for gag or pharyngeal reflex include gloves, tongue depressor and a source of light sufficient to illuminate the back of the mouth. Ask the patient if you can see inside his/her mouth. Ask the patient to open the mouth as wide as possible and say 'Ahh' or yawn. Using the tongue depressor, push down on the tongue. Observe how the structures in the oral cavity move involuntarily. The soft palate should rise symmetrically and the uvula remained midline. Next, firmly press the tongue depressor around the midpoint of the arched tongue to see of the patient gags. Refer to Figures 7.21.-7.22.

Clinical Nutrition Pearls: Oral Assessment

Diseases and disorders associated with chew and swallowing are medical diagnoses. Failure to recognize changes in the oral cavity can result in serious consequences. Continuation of current intervention strategies or inappropriate intervention strategies can create additional problems for the adult with declining nutrition status. Mealtime observation followed by assessment of specific cranial nerves may reveal physiological changes that have been overlooked. Work collaboratively with the speech and language pathologist or swallowing therapist to determine the most appropriate food and beverage consistency. Appropriate nutrition diagnoses may include suboptimal or excessive intake, changes in functional status specific to swallowing, biting or chewing and behavioral-environmental issues specific to knowledge, beliefs or physical activity and function. Collaborate with other healthcare team members to identify changes in speaking and swallowing.

Figures 7.19.-7.20 Assessment for Cranial Nerves I & V

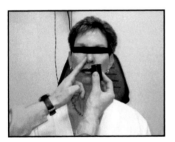
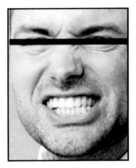

Figures 7.21.-7.22. Assessment for Cranial Nerves IX & X
Gag Reflex or Pharyngeal Reflex

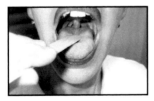
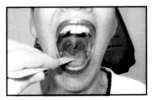

Abdominal Exam

An abdominal examination is a common procedure done by physicians, physician assistants, nurse practitioners and nurses. This is a skill that RDNs can learn to do if applicable in the practice setting. Remember that the purpose of doing the abdominal examination is to gather data to support nutrition diagnoses and to monitor and evaluate the effectiveness of nutrition interventions. The abdominal exam involves inspection, auscultation percussion and palpation.

The abdomen is divided into four quadrants. By using two imaginary lines that intersect at the navel, visually divide the abdomen into right upper quadrant (RUQ), right lower quadrant (RLQ), left upper quadrant (LUQ) and lower left quadrant (LLQ).

Each quadrant contains important organs and knowing where they are in quadrants may make a difference in your assessment. If the patient complains of abdominal pain, be sure to evaluate this area last or consult another healthcare team member before proceeding with the abdominal examination. Table 7.3. notes the organs approximate location in each quadrant.

Practical Applications for NFPA: Abdominal Exam

To conduct and abdominal examination, the assessor needs good light, stethoscope and a relaxed, well-draped patient in the supine position. Close the door to the room and draw the curtains around the bed to ensure privacy. Explain the type of exam that you would like to conduct and obtain consent from the patient or authorized representative. Even if the patient is unable to communication, it is important to speak to them, introduce yourself and explain what you are planning to do and explain each step through the process. The patient/resident may be able to hear and understand the information you are sharing yet unable to respond.

Make sure the patient is comfortable and relaxed having a pillow for the head and knees. Ask the patient to keep the arms at the sides or folded across the chest. Check that the patient has an empty bladder. The patient must be draped properly for this exam. The abdomen is exposed from just above the xiphoid process to the symphysis pubis. The groin should be visible, but the genitalia draped.

Table 7.3. Organs & GI Structures by Abdominal Quadrant

RUQ	LUQ
gallbladder	spleen
head of pancreas	body of pancreas
liver	L lobe of liver
pylorus	stomach
duodenum	L portion kidney
R adrenal gland	L adrenal gland
portion R kidney	splenic flexure of colon
hepatic flexure of colon, portion of ascending and transverse colon	

RLQ	LLQ
appendix	lower L kidney
lower R kidney	sigmoid colon
cecum	portion of descending colon
portion of ascending colon	bladder (if distended)
ovary and salpinx	ovary and salpinx
uterus (if enlarged)	uterus (if enlarged)
bladder (if distended)	L ureter
R ureter	

Begin the exam by asking some questions to better understand the medical concerns and determine any omissions in the health history.

Ask questions specific to abdominal pain such as:
• Are you having any abdominal pain or tenderness?
• Please show me where you are having pain.
• Describe the pain (piercing, dull, burning, crampy)
• How would you rate the pain on a 10 point scale with 0 as pain-free and 10 being the worst pain you could imagine?
• Is the pain constant or does it come and go?
• Is the pain worse with eating? If yes, ask how long after eating does the pain start or worsen?
• Is the pain lessened or worse after having a bowel movement?
• Are you taking aspirin, acetaminophen , steroid or NSAIDS?

Ask questions specific to GI symptoms such as:
Have your eating habits changed recently? In what way?
Have you had any nausea or vomiting?
• Do you have any abdominal distention or feel bloated?
• Do certain foods upset your stomach, give you heartburn, reflux or excessive belching?
• Are you experiencing early satiety, altered taste or poor appetite?

Ask questions specific to bowel habits such as:
• Have you had any changes in bowel habits?
• Flatus?
• Constipation?
• Diarrhea?
• When was your last bowel movement? Describe the color, consistency, presence of blood.

For ostomy patients only
- What is the volume of output or number of times you have to empty ostomy bag?
- When was the last time you emptied ostomy bag?
Describe the color, consistency, presence of blood.

Inspection

Begin the exam by inspecting the surface and movement of the abdomen. Note the contours of the abdomen, i.e. flat, round, protuberant or scaphoid. A healthy adult has a flat or slightly round abdomen. A scaphoid or concave abdomen may suggest loss of subcutaneous fat due to suboptimal energy intake or malnutrition. A protuberant abdomen may suggest a number of problems noted on Table 7.4. Note any visible organs or masses that extend below the rib cage.

Table 7.4. Six F's of Abdominal Distention

Sign	Possible Etiology
fluid	ascites
fat	obesity
flatulence	gas
fetus	pregnancy
feces	constipation
full-sized tumor	abnormal lesion

If you suspect abdominal distention, ask the patient if he/she feels bloated or distended. It is important to differentiate between obesity and abdominal distention. Abdominal distention feels firmer than a non-distended obese abdomen. Consult with other members of the healthcare team if your findings are atypical.

Also observe for non-healing wounds. Poor wound healing may be due to insufficient energy and or protein intake.

Review the Nutrition Prescription and intake data to determine if additional nutrients are needed. Note the appearance of the wound dressing. It should be clean and dry without drainages, blood or odor. Alert the wound care nurse if you have concerns.

If the patient has a nutrition support access device i.e. percutaneous endoscopic gastrostomy site or peripherally inserted central catheter exit site, check for signs of infection, signs of malfunction or malposition. Inspect the skin around the device for erythema, swelling or drainage. Also check drains, fistulas or ostomies for signs of drainage, infection or malposition. Consult with other members of the healthcare team if you have concerns.

Auscultation
Next, listen for bowel sounds. This is done before percussion and palpation because these techniques may increase peristalsis and interfere with normal sounds. Be sure that your hands and stethoscope are warm. Approach the patient calmly and avoid quick movements. Watch the patient's face for signs of pain or discomfort.

Place the diaphragm of the stethoscope gently on the abdomen at the right lower quadrant for 2-5 minutes or until you hear bowel sounds. This is the location of the ileocecal valve. Check the other quadrants if sounds are not heard at the right lower quadrant. Since bowel sounds are transmitted throughout the abdomen, listening at the right lower quadrant is often sufficient. However some clinicians listen for 1 to 2 minutes in each quadrant.

The healthy patient will have gurgling sounds made by the movement of intestines as they push food through the gut.

The intestines are hollow, like water pipes, and sounds echo through the abdomen. Normal sounds consist of clicks and gurgles that occur between 5-43 per minute. Occasionally you will hear borborygmi or prolonged gurgles of hyperperistalas i.e. 'stomach growling.' These bowel sounds may be audible without the stethoscope!

The gut is hypoactive during sleep and after surgery. Hypoactive bowel sounds are quieter and less frequent than normal bowel sounds. If you do not hear anything for 3 to 5 minutes of listening for bowel sounds at any of the quadrants, hypoactive bowel signs or absent bowel sounds should be documented. This may suggest ileus, peritonitis or the gut is not working following surgery or constipation. Alert members of the healthcare team of abnormal findings for confirmation.

Learning to interpret bowel sounds takes practice. If you have never listened to bowel sounds before, there are numerous resources on the Internet to listen to normal bowel sounds. Once you have familiarized yourself with common bowel sounds, practice auscultation until your are thoroughly familiar with variations in bowel sounds.

Percussion

The third step is percussion. This technique helps detect the presence of gaseous distention, fluid or solid masses. Always ask the patient to point out areas of pain in order to avoid percussing them. Percuss the abdomen lightly in all four quadrants to assess the distribution of tympany and dullness. Tympany usually predominates because of gases in the GI tract. Scattered area of dullness from fluid or feces is also typical. Consult with members of the healthcare team if you have concerns.

Learning to interpret percussion sounds takes practice. If you have never listened to the different sounds before, there are numerous resources on the Internet to listen to tympany and dull sounds. Once you have familiarized yourself with the difference in tympany and dull sounds, practice percussion until your are thoroughly familiar with variations in sounds.

Palpation

The next step is light palpation to assess for tenderness, muscular resistance, and superficial organs and masses. Keep your hand and forearm on a horizontal plane over the abdomen and keep with fingers together. Lightly press in about 0.75 inch for each palpations in all quadrants. Be sure to raise your hand off the skin when moving from one quadrant to another. Note any signs of discomfort and report findings to other healthcare team members. Do not palpitate the abdomen if the patient has had abdominal surgery, trauma, peritonitis or if there is anything questionable about the abdominal status.

Clinical Nutrition Pearls: Abdominal Exam

Diseases and disorders of the digestive system are medical diagnoses. Appropriate nutrition diagnoses may include altered gastrointestinal function, altered nutrient utilization, or intake specific criteria. Failure to recognize changes in the digestive system or problems related to nutrition support devices can result in serious consequences. Continuation of current intervention strategies or inappropriate intervention strategies can create additional problems for the adult with declining nutrition status. Individuals with malabsorptive disorders or who have had weight loss surgery are at risk for a variety of nutrient deficiencies noted on Table 7.5. Always collaborate with other medical team members to determine the etiology of digestive system concerns.

Table 7.5. Nutrient Deficiencies Reported in Malabsorptive Disorders & Weight Loss Surgery

Nutrient	Deficiency Signs/Symptoms
Essential Fatty Acid	Xerosis of skin
Iron	Fatigue, pallor, koilonychia
Vitamin A	Xerosis of skin & eyes, follicular hyperkeratosis, night blindness or impaired night vision, Bitot's spots, hazy dry softened cornea
Vitamin B12	Pernicious anemia, tingling or numbness in hands & feet, impaired cognitive status
Vitamin D	↓ 25(OH)D, ↑ risk for falls, fractures & functional decline
Vitamin K	↑ bleeding times
Thiamin	↓ Stores due to prolonged vomiting, neurological changes
Zinc	Delayed wound healing, dermatitis

Figures 7.23.-7.24. illustrate techniques used in the abdominal assessment.

Figure 7.23. Palpation   **Figure 7.24.** Auscultation

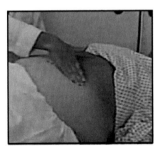
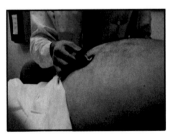

Figure 7.25. Abdominal Quadrants

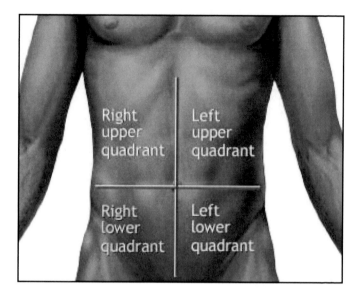

Figures 7.26-7.27. Signs of Infection

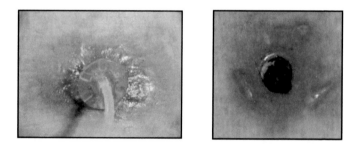

References

Aills L, Blankenship J, Buffington C, et al. ASMBS allied health nutritional guidelines for the surgical weight loss patient. Surg Obes Relat Dis. 2008;4(Supp):73S–108S.

Aasheim ET. Night blindness after duodenal switch. Surg Obes Relat Dis. 2008;4(5):685-6

Aasheim ET. Vitamin status after bariatric surgery: a randomized study of gastric bypass and duodenal switch. Am J Clin Nutr 2009:1;15 -22

Aasheim ET. Wernicke encephalopathy after bariatric surgery. A systematic review. Ann Surg. 2005;248(5):714–20

Bickley,L. Bates guide to physical examination, 10th ed. Philadelphia,PA: Lippincott, 2009.

Bloomberg, R.D., Fleishman, A., Nalle, J.E. et al. (2005) Nutritional deficiencies following bariatric surgery: what have we learned? Obesity Surgery, 15, 145–154.

Bourdel-Marchasson I, Barateau M (2000)A multi-center trial of the effects of oral nutritional supplementation in critically ill older inpatients. Nutrition. 16: 1-5.

CMS: MDS 3.0 for Nursing Home. http://www.cms.gov/NursingHomeQualityInits/30_NHQIMDS30TechnicalInformation.asp#Top OfPage.htm. Accessed November 17, 2011.

Gehrer S. Fewer nutrient deficiencies after laparoscopic sleeve gastrectomy (LSG) than after laparoscopic Roux-Y-gastric bypass (LRYGB)-a prospective study. Obes Surg. 2010 Apr;20(4):447-53. Epub 2010 Jan 26.

Gollobin C. Bariatric beriberi. Obes Surg. 2002;12:309–311.

Hakeam HA. Impact of laparoscopic sleeve gastrectomy on iron indices: 1 year follow-up. Obes Surg. 2009 Nov;19(11):1491-6.

Juhasz-Pocsine K. Neurological complications of gastric bypass surgery for morbid obesity. Neurology. 2007;68:1843–1850.

Lakhani SV, Shah HN, Alexander K. Small intestinal bacterial overgrowth and thiamine deficiency after Roux-en-Y gastric bypass surgery in obese patients. Nutr Res. 2008 May;28(5):293-8.

Madan, A.K., Orth, W.S., Tichansky, D.S. et al. (2006) Vitamin and trace mineral levels after laparoscopic gastric bypass. Obesity Surgery, 16, 603–606.

Mahowald JM.(1981) Hypernatremia in the elderly: relation to infection and mortality. JAGS ;29:177-80.

Makarewicz W. Wernicke's syndrome after sleeve gastrectomy. Obes Surg. 2007 May;17(5):704-6.

Moccia, L Abdominal examinations: A guide for dietitians. DNS Support Line.Apriol 201133(2), 16-21.

Oh, Robert C. Vitamin B12 Deficiency. American Family Physician. Vol 67, number 5 / March 1, 2003.

Poitou Bernert, C., Ciangura, C.(2007) Nutritional deficiency after gastric bypass: diagnosis, prevention and treatment. Diabetes and Metabolism, 33, 13–24. Epub 2007 January 26.

Shikora SA, Kim JJ, Tarnoff ME. Nutrition and gastrointestinal complications of bariatric surgery. Nutr Clin Pract. 2007 Feb;22(1):29-40. Review.

Shilen V. Small intestinal bacterial overgrowth and thiamine deficiency after Roux-en-Y gastric bypass surgery in obese patients. Nutrition Research. Volume 28, Issue 5, May 2008, 293-298.

Snyder-Marlow G. Nutrition care for patients undergoing laparoscopic sleeve gastrectomy for weight loss. J Am Diet Assoc. 2010 Apr;110(4):600-7.

Strain GW. Comparison of weight loss and body composition changes with four surgical procedures. Surg Obes Relat Dis. 2009 Sep-Oct;5(5):582-7.

Toh SY, Zarshenas N Prevalence of nutrient deficiencies in bariatric patients. Nutrition. 2009 Nov-Dec;25(11-12):1150-6.

Vargas-Ruiz, A.G. (2008) Prevalence of iron, folate, and vitamin B12 deficiency anemia after laparoscopic Roux-en-Y gastric bypass. Obesity Surgery, 18, 288–293. Epub 2008 January 23.

Vitamin B-12 Associated Neurological Diseases http://emedicine.medscape.com/article/1152670-overview

Chapter 8
Tools for Assessing Bone Health

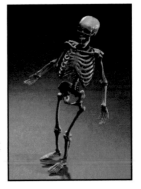

Vitamin D, calcium, magnesium and vitamin K are the primary nutrients associated with bone health. Significant changes in normal growth and development of bones occurs with a vitamin D deficiency.

In the 1640s physicians noted that children living in the inner cities had growth retardation, skeletal deformities, rachitic rosary (bony projections along the rib cage) and either bowed legs or knocked knees compared to healthy children. The disorder was called rickets derived from the old English word 'wrickken', meaning to twist or bend. In addition, vitamin D deficiency causes disruption in chondrocyte maturation at the ephyseal plates, leading to widening of the ends of long bones and costochondral junctions. Refer to Figures 8.1.-8.2.

Figure 8.1. Rickets vs. Normal Growth (child in middle)

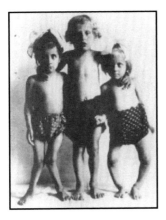

Figure 8.2 Rachitic Rosary

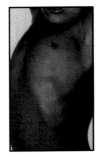

Rickets were common in children living in polluted inner cities of Europe and northeastern United States by from the 1600s to the early 1900s. The relationship between sunshine and rickets was recognized by the early 1920s. Once vitamin D was identifed and added to selected foods, rickets were essentially eradicated.

However, in the 21st century, vitamin D deficiency has emerged in all age groups due to insufficient exposure to sunlight and insufficient dietary intake of vitamin D. The role of vitamin D and calcium in maintaining healthy bones is clear in the scientific literature. There is emerging research demonstrating a greater role of vitamin D in risk reduction for falls, fractures, functional decline and many chronic and autoimmune diseases.

Vitamin D deficiency has more subtle effects on the skeleton of adults than on children. Secondary hyperparathyroidism mobilizes calcium from the skeleton and reduces bone mineral density. A reduction in bone mineral density may precipitate or exacerbate osteoporosis. Osteoporosis is a chronic progressive disease of multifactorial etiology characterized by low bone mass and loss of bone tissue that may lead to weak and fragile bones. It is the most common metabolic bone disease in the United States primarily in postmenopausal women of Caucasian or Asian decent. It does occur in both sexes, all races, and all age groups. The disease often does not become clinically apparent until a fracture occurs. Loss of height and kyphosis or a curve in the spine are common with osteoporosis. These skeletal changes occur following several vertebral fractures or compression fractures and can be defined using the occiput-wall test. Kyphosis in females over the age of 65 has been identified as a marker of poor physical function (Antonelli-Incalzi, 2007).

A vitamin D deficiency affects the strength of the collagen matrix of bone critical for structural support. The abnormal collagen matrix expands on the periosteal covering, which is innervated with sensory pain fibers. The clinical consequence is people with osteomalacia experience aching in their bones (Malabana, 1998; Gloth, 1991). Osteomalacia is also associated with muscle aches and if often misdiagnosed as fibromyalgia, chronic fatigue syndrome or other nonspecific collagen vascular diseases. It is estimated that 40-60 % of patients with fibromyalgia may have a vitamin D deficiency and osteomalacia (Holick, 2004). Glerup (2000) reported that 88 % of Danish Arab women with muscle weakness and pain were vitamin D deficient. More than 90 % of children and adults aged 10-65 years complaining of nonspecific pain, muscle and bone aches at a Minnesota hospital were found to be vitamin D deficient (Plotnikoff, 2003). Lower concentrations of serum 25(OH) D were associated with increased risk of moderate to severe back pain in older women, but not men (Hicks, 2008).

It is estimated that 60-80% of pre-operative weight loss surgery patients are vitamin D deficient. Buffington (1993) reported an increased prevalence of low vitamin D with severe obesity and a negative correlation between BMI and vitamin D levels. Vitamin D deficiency has been reported in 32% of sleeve gastrectomy patients (Gehrer, 2010).

Vitamin D toxicity is rare. It is discussed in Chapter 9.

NFPA for a vitamin D deficiency or for osteoporosis begins with a review of the medical history for risk factors, recent fractures, diagnosis of chronic fatigue syndrome or fibromyalgia. In addition to race, age and gender, other risk factors include family history, small body frame, a diet low in calcium, history of anorexia nervosa, smoking, sedentary lifestyle, and excessive alcohol consumption. Observe posture and early signs of a kyphosis. Some questions to consider include:

- Have you lost height over time?
- Do you recall if your mother or grandmother lost height over time?
- Do you have frequent muscle ache? If yes, ask how often?
- Tell me about your recent fracture.
- Was this a trauma fracture? Did you fall?
- How many times have you fallen in the last month?
- Do you recall if other adult women in your family have experienced broken bones?
- Do you take vitamin mineral supplements? If yes, what type?
- How much sun exposure do you receive daily during the summer months? Do you use sun screen?

Practical Applications for NFPA: Bone Health
Bone health can be assessed using family history of osteoporosis, health history that includes fractures, laboratory test results for serum 25(OH)D, anthropometric data, medications associated with bone loss are noted on Table 8.1, dietary intake data, and other radiography studies. Other nutrient deficiencies associated with osteoporosis are noted on table 8.2.

Lifestyle choices including smoking, inactivity and high alcohol consumption also increase risk for osteoporosis. Medical conditions associated with vitamin D deficiency and osteoporosis are noted on Table 8.3.

The gold standard for assessing bone mass density and assessing bone fracture risk is dual-energy X-ray absorptiometry (DXA). Recent developments in DXA

Table 8.1. Medications Associated with Accelerated Bone Loss

Anticonvulsants - Phenytoin, barbiturates, carbamazepine
Antipsychotic drugs
Antiretroviral drugs
Aromatase inhibitors - Exemestane, anastrozole
Chemotherapeutic/transplant drugs - Cyclosporine, tacrolimus, platinum compounds, cyclophosphamide, ifosfamide, methotrexate
Furosemide
Glucocorticoids and corticotropin (> 3 month use)
Heparin (long-term)
Hormonal/endocrine therapies - Gonadotropin-releasing hormone (GnRH) agonists, luteinizing hormone-releasing hormone (LHRH) analogs, depomedroxyprogesterone, excessive thyroid supplementation
Lithium
Selective serotonin reuptake inhibitors

Table 8.2. Nutrient Deficiencies Associated with Osteoporosis

calcium	vitamin K
magnesium	protein
vitamin D	

Table 8.3. Nutrition-Related Conditions Associated with Osteoporosis

bariatric surgery	malnutrition
celiac disease	parenteral nutrition
gastrectomy	primary biliary cirrhosis
malabsorption	

enable images of the whole spine to be obtained allowing for diagnosis of vertebral fractures. The DXA scan can detect bone loss after about a 1 % loss compared to a 40 % loss using a standard x-ray. The results are either T-scores or Z-scores plus the standard deviation (SD). One SD equals about 10-15 % bone loss in young adults. The Z-score looks at loss compared to the average bone density for the patient's age. The T-score looks at bone loss compared to young adults aged 25-45 years. The World Health Organization (WHO) definitions for skeletal health using bone mass density are noted in Table 8.4.

Table 8.4. Skeletal Health Definitions Using Bone Mass Density

Category	Definition
Normal	less than 1 SD below norms
Osteopenia	greater than 1 SD and less than 2.5 SD below norms
Osteoporosis	2.5 SD below norms
Severe Osteoporosis	greater than 2.5 SD below norms

Key: SD- standard deviation

Figure 8.3. Normal Bone   **Figure 8.4.** Osteoporosis

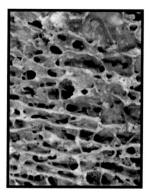
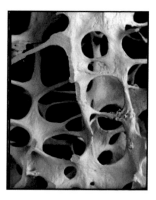

Other risk assessment tools to estimate risk for declining bone health include the wall occiput test and the rib pelvis distance test. The occiput-wall distance, a measure of kyphosis, has been associated with postural instability, osteoporosis, disability, depression and reduced physical function (i.e. walking and climbing stairs) (Antonelli-Incalzi,

2007; Tribus, 1998; Balzini, 2003; Di Bari, 2004; Kado, 2005; Ryan, 1997). Vitamin D insufficiency and deficiency have been associated with increased risk for falls, fractures and functional declines (Bischoll, 2004).

The wall occiput test involves having the patient/resident stand as straight as possible against a wall or flat surface. Measure the distance between the back of the head (occiput) and the wall. A positive test is defined in JAMA (Green, 2004) as greater than zero. The Osteoporosis Society of Canada defines a positive test as greater than 6 cm (Siminoski, 2006). Refer to Figure 8.7.

The rib-pelvis distance test measures the distance between the bottom of the rib cage and the top of the pelvis bone. Normal skeletal health is defined as less than or equal to two fingerbreadths or 3.6 cm (Green, 2004). Refer to Figure 8.8.

WHO fracture-risk algorithm FRAX, was developed to calculate the 10-year probability of a hip fracture and the 10-year probability of any major osteoporotic fracture (i.e. clinical spine, hip, forearm, or humerus fracture) in a given patient. These calculations account for femoral neck bone mineral density (BMD) and other clinical risk factors including age, gender, history of fracture, low BMI, history or conditions associated with secondary osteoporosis, parental history of hip fracture, smoking, alcohol intake. FRAX algorithm is useful in identifying patients in the osteopenic range who are most likely to benefit from treatment.

Clinical Nutrition Pearls: Bone Health

Criteria to define vitamin D insufficiency and deficiency are controversial. The 2011 recommendations of the Institute of Medicine for the DRI for vitamin D were set based on a different cutpoint for serum 25(OH)D that was recommend by WHO and many researchers. The International Osteoporosis Foundations released their recommendations in 2010 as well. To date, these organizations do not agree on the criteria defining vitamin D sufficiency, insufficiency and deficiency. The current criteria by organization is noted in Table 8.5.

Table 8.5. Criteria for Defining Vitamin D Status by Organization

Organization	Deficiency; Rickets or Osteomalacia	Insufficiency	Sufficiency
WHO	< 50 nmol/L; < 20 ng/mL	50-80 nmol/L; 20-32 ng/mL	>80 nmol/L; >32 ng/mL
IOF	No cut point	No cutpoint	>75 nmol/L; >30 ng/mL
2011 IOM, DRI provides sufficient levels to achieve these cutpoints	Adults < 30 nmol/L; < 12 ng/mL Infant/Child < 27 nmol/L; < 11 ng/mL	No cutpoint	>30 nmol/L; > 12 ng/mL

Diagnosing early changes in bone density in females during the menopausal transition or postmenopausal using a DXA scan has been recommended for women with one or more risk factors. Individuals with low bone density or osteopenia are candidates for pharmacological interventions.

As part of healthcare reform in the United States (US), the benefit of these costly tests has been reviewed by the US Preventive Services Task Force (USPSTF). The USPSTF recommends screening for osteoporosis in women aged 65 years or older. In younger women screening is recommended for those whose fracture risk is equal to or greater than that of a 65-yr-old white woman who has no additional risk factors. The USPSTF concludes that the current evidence is insufficient to assess the balance of benefits and harms of screening for osteoporosis in men. In light of these recommendations, it is likely that fewer DXA scans will be available and alternate assessment tools will be utilized.

Vitamin D deficiency, rickets, adult rickets, low bone density and osteoporosis are all medical diagnoses. Nutrition diagnoses that may apply include suboptimal calcium intake, suboptimal vitamin D intake, altered gastrointestinal function, food-medication interaction or altered nutrient utilization. Failure to recognize changes in bone health can result in serious consequences. Always collaborate with other medical team members to determine the etiology of declining bone health.

Figure 8.5. Affect of Aging on Spine

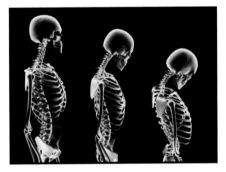

Figure 8.6. Kyphosis

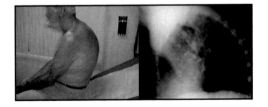

Figure 8.7. Wall-Occiput Test   **Figure 8.8.** Rib-Pelvis Test

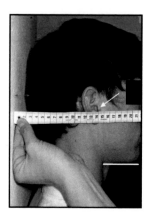
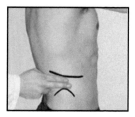

References

Ahmed SF, Elmantaser M. Secondary osteoporosis. Endocr Dev. 2009;16:170-90.

AACE medical guidelines for clinical practice for the prevention & treatment of postmenopausal osteoporosis: 2001 ed, with selected updates for 2003. Endocr Pract. Nov-Dec 2003;9(6):544-64.

Anotnelli-Incalzi, R. Relationship between the occiput-wall distance and physical performance in the elderly: a cross sectional study. 2007 Aging Clin Exp Res 19(3)207-212.

Balsa JA. Chronic increase of bone turnover markers after BPD is related to secondary hyperparathyroidism & weight loss. Relation with bone mineral density. Obes Surg. 2010 Apr;20(4):468-73.

Balzini L. Clinical characteristics of flexed posture in elderly women. J Am Geriatr Soc. 2003;51:1419–26.

Bischoff-Ferrari HA. Prevention of nonvertebral fractures with oral vitamin D & dose dependency: meta-analysis of randomized controlled trials. Arch Intern Med. Mar 23 2009;169(6):551-61.

Bischoff-Ferrari, HA(2004) Effect of vitamin D on falls: a meta-analysis. JAMA; 291(16): 1999-2006.

Clinician's Guide to Prevention and Treatment of Osteoporosis. Washington, DC: National Osteoporosis Foundation; 2008.

Chapuy MC, Preziosi P(1997) Prevalence of vitamin D insufficiency in an adult normal population. Osteoporosis Int 7(5): 439-43.

Dawson-Hughes B. (1997) Effect of calcium & vitamin D supplementation on bone density in men & women 65 yrs of age or older. NEJM ; 337(10): 670-6

Di Bari M. Thoracic kyphosis and ventilatory dysfunction in unselected older persons: an epidemiological study in Dicomano, Italy. J Am Geriatr Soc. 2004;52:909–15.

Vitamin D Individual Patient Analysis of Randomized Trials. Patient level pooled analysis of 68 500 patients from 7 major vitamin D fracture trials in US & Europe. BMJ. Jan 12 2010;340:b5463.

Glerup,H, Mikkelsen, K et al (2000)Commonly recommended daily intake of vitamin D is not sufficient if sunlight exposure is limited. J Intern Med 247:260-8.

Gloth FM III, Gundberg CM, Hollis BW,(1995) Vitamin D deficiency in homebound elderly persons. JAMA 1995; 274(21): 1683-6

Green, A, Colón-Emeric,C (2004) Does this woman have osteoporosis? JAMA; 292:2890-2900.

Hicks, G, Ferrucci, L (2008) Associations between vitamin D status and pain in older adults. The Invecchiare in Chianti Study. JAGS, March 5 e-pub.

Holick MF. Vitamin D. Importance in the prevention of cancers, type 1 diabetes, heart disease, & osteoporosis. AJClN 2004; 79:362-371.

Holick, MF (2004) Sunlight and vitamin D for bone health and prevention of autoimmune disease, cancers and cardiovascular disease. AJCN 80(supp) 1678S-88S.

Kado DM. Hyperkyphotic posture and poor physical functional ability in older community-dwelling men and women. J Gerontol. 2005;60:633–7.

Kanis JA. Assessment of fracture risk and its application to screening for postmenopausal osteoporosis: synopsis of a WHO report. WHO Study Group. Osteoporos Int. Nov 1994;4(6):368-81.

Kanis JA, McCloskey EV, 3rd, Khaltaev N. A reference standard for the description of osteoporosis. Bone. Mar 2008;42(3):467-75.

Majumdar SR, Lier DA. Osteoporosis case manager for patients with hip fractures: results of a cost-effectiveness analysis conducted alongside a randomized trial. Arch Intern Med. Jan 12 2009;169(1):25-31.

Malabana, AO, Turner, AK, Holick, MF(1998) Severe generalized bone pain and osteoporosis in a premenopausal black female: effect of vitamin D replacement. J Clin Densitometr 1:201-4.

National Osteoporosis Foundation. Clinician's Guide to Prevention and Treatment of Osteoporosis. Available at http://www.nof. org/professionals/clinical-guidelines. Accessed November, 2011.

Plotnikoff, GA, Quigley, JM. (2003)Prevalence of severe hypovitaminosis D in patients with persistent nonspecific musculoskeletal pain. Mayo Clin Proc. 78:1463-70.

Ryan SD, Fried LP. The impact of kyphosis on daily functioning. J Am Geriatr Soc. 1997;45:1479–86

Siminoski, K (2005) Vertebral compression fractures: practical tips for effective assessment. Osteoporosis Update 9(1) 4-5, Osteoporosis Society of Canada.

Tribus CB. Scheuermann's kyphosis in adolescents and adults: diagnosis and management. J Am Acad Orthop Surg. 1998;6:36–43.

U.S. Preventive Services Task Force. Screening for Osteoporosis: U.S. Preventive Services Task Force Recommendation Statement. Ann Intern Med. December, 2011.

World Health Organization Fracture Risk Assessment Tool. Available at http://www.shef.ac.uk/FRAX/. Accessed December, 2011.

Chapter 9
Tools for Assessing
HEENT
&
Nutrition-Related Conditions

HEENT stands for head, eyes, ears, nose and throat. Changes in HEENT are often medical diagnoses or may be related to misuse of medications. However, changes may also be due to nutrient deficiencies or toxicities that are overlooked by the medical team. NFPA is a vital tool to correlate changes in HEENT with suboptimal nutrient intakes or megadoses of selected nutrients. In previous chapters some aspects of the assessment of the HEENT have already been discussed (i.e. cranial nerves) and will not be repeated.

The decision to initiate NFPA of the HEENT and assess for nutrition-related conditions is triggered by data in the medical record or information gathered during the interview. Some data to note include a change in frequency and/or type of headaches, change in vision, vertigo, increased fatigue, disequilibrium, changes in temperature tolerance, and unplanned weight loss or gain. Some questions to consider in assessing for changes in HEENT and nutrition-related conditions include:

Head and Headaches
• Your medical record indicates that you are having more frequent headaches. Have your headaches changed in severity recently?
• Do you experience nausea or vomiting after the onset of the headache?

• Do you think that certain foods trigger the headache?
• Have you changed your eating habits recently?
• Do you have any food sensitivities or allergies?
• Do you take vitamin mineral supplements daily? If yes, what type and dosage.
• Do you take herbal supplements daily? If yes, what type and dosage.

Eyes
• How is your vision?
• Have you had any changes in your eyes or with your vision?
• Do you have any difficulty seeing at night?
• Do your eyes feel dry?
• It is difficult to open your eyes when you wake up?

Ears
• How is your hearing?
• Do you have episodes of dizziness or disequilibrium?

Nose
• How is your sense of smell?
• Has your sense of smell changed recently?

Mouth, Throat & Neck
• Have you noticed any swollen gland or lumps in your neck?
• Do you dress more warmly or less warmly than other people?
• Have your eating patterns (types of food) changed over the last week or months?
• Has the amount of food eaten changed?
• Any changes with chewing or swallowing foods?

Lipid Soluble Vitamins

The lipid soluble vitamins include vitamins A, D, E and K. These compounds are soluble in lipid solvents and are absorbed along with dietary fats. They are not normally excreted in the urine and tend to be stored in the body in moderate amounts.

Deficiencies of lipid soluble vitamins are rare in healthy adults who eat a variety of foods or who take multiple vitamin supplements because of the body stores. Individuals following restrictive diets and those with malabsorptive conditions are at risk for lipid soluble vitamin deficiencies. Toxicities are primarily from chronic intakes of large doses of individual vitamins.

Vitamin A

The major sources of vitamin A in the diet are provitamin A carotenoids founds in fruits and vegetables and retinyl esters found in animal products. Vitamin supplements may contain either or both forms of vitamin A. The absorption of vitamin A either as preformed vitamin A (retinol) or provitamin A carotenoids is a complex process that is not fully understood in healthy adults or in patients with compromised digestive systems.

The bioavailability of retinol is generally more than 80%, whereas the bioavailability and bioconversion of carotenes are lower. Factors that increase absorption of carotenoids in the duodenum are the presence of a minimum of 3-5 g fat and low pH. However, studies of carotenoid absorption in patients whose duodenum has been surgically bypassed (i.e. high pH) demonstrate an increase in serum retinol concentrations. This clinical finding suggests that the absorption of provitamin A may be due to passive diffusion throughout the small intestine. It also suggests that for the patients with malabsorptive conditions, the formula used to convert mcg beta-carotene to mcg retinol is unrepresentative of actual utilization (12 mcg beta-carotene= 1 mcg retinol).

Vitamin A Deficiency

Vitamin A deficiency is endemic in countries where the staple foods are devoid of beta-carotene due to prolonged dietary deprivation. In developed countries, a secondary vitamin A deficiency may be due to decreased bioavailability of provitamin A carotenoids or to interference with absorption, storage, or transport of vitamin A. Deficiencies have has been reported in adults with malabsorptive disorders, cystic fibrosis, Whipple's disease, tropical sprue, celiac disease, bacterial overgrowth in the intestines, pancreatic disease, cholestasis, inflammatory bowel disease, cirrhosis of the liver, bile duct obstruction and amyloidosis. In addition, vitamin A insufficiency or deficiency several years following weight loss surgery is reported in up to one third of patients having had a Roux-en-Y procedure (Madan, 2006; Aasheim, 2009) and half of those who had the biliopancreatic diversion procedure (Dolan, 2004; Scopinaro, 1998). Researchers theorize that the useable small intestine may not provide sufficient absorptive surfaces or that the diet does not contain sufficient fat or that the diet does not include sufficient amounts of vitamin A from food and supplements. The need for higher intakes of preformed vitamin A retinol may be required for these patients to maintain sufficient vitamin A stores.

Sub-optimal intakes of zinc and iron may compound a vitamin A deficiency due to metabolic interrelationships among these nutrients. In developing countries, a decreased resistance to infections and increased incidence of nutrition-related anemia is associated with a vitamin A deficiency. In zinc deficiency, impaired synthesis of retinol binding protein (RBP) occurs. The short half-life of RBP compounded by reduced synthesis affects retinol transport by RBP from the liver to the circulation and to other tissues. The mechanism by which iron affects vitamin A metabolism has not been identified, but randomized, double-blind studies have shown that vitamin A supplementation alone is not sufficient to improve vitamin A deficiency in the presence of coexisting iron deficiency (Munoz, 2000; Jimenez,2009).

In addition, alcohol affects the metabolism of vitamin A. Alcohol dehydrogenase catalyzes the conversion of retinol to retinaldehyde, which is then oxidized to retinoic acid. The affinity of alcohol dehydrogenase to ethanol impedes the conversion of retinol to retinoic acid.

Early signs of a vitamin A deficiency include changes in the eyes, skin, hair, nails and pruritus (itching). Ocular changes begin as chronic dry eye (that is not medication related). As the deficiency worsens, conjunctival xerosis, corneal xerosis, impaired night vision and nyctalopia (difficulty adjusting from light to dark environments or night blindness) are evident. Cutaneous changes include dry skin leading to dermatitis, follicular hyperkeratosis (goose flesh), dry hair, and brittle nails.

As the vitamin A deficiency advances, additional ocular changes include keratomalacia, Bitot's spots may appear on the sclera, and the cornea may harden and scar. Ocular changes ultimately lead to permanent blindness. Refer to Figures 9.1.-9.5.

Hypervitaminosis A: Vitamin A Toxicity

Individuals consuming excessive amounts of vitamin A precursors in food, mainly carrots, may develop carotenemia. It is manifested by a yellow-orange coloring of the skin, primarily on the palms of the hands and the soles of the feet. Carotene is a lipochrome that normally adds yellow color to the skin. With elevated blood levels of carotene, the prominence of this yellowing is increased. Red hues may be from pigments such as carotenoids, porphyrins, turacin, pheomelanin, psittacofulvins, and hemoglobin (Toral, 2008). It differs from jaundice in that the sclera remain white. Carotenemia may also be associated with the ingestion of carotene-rich nutritional supplements (Takita, 2006; Schwartz, 2011). Other than the cosmetic effect, carotenemia has no adverse consequences because the conversion of carotenes to retinol is not sufficient to cause toxicity. Refer Figure 9.6.

Excessive intakes of preformed vitamin A (retinol) have been shown to have adverse skeletal effects in both animal models and clinical trials (Togari, 1991; Scheven, 1990; Abu-Hijleh, 1997). In humans, chronic vitamin A toxicity can cause hypercalcemia (Frame, 1974), impaired bone remodeling, and bone abnormalities (Hathcock, 1990; Bendich, 1989). In addition, high intake of synthetic retinoids has been associated with decreased bone mass (Okada, 1994; DiGiovanna, 1995) and suppressed biochemical markers of bone turnover (Kindmark, 1998).

However, data from the Women's Health Initiative Observational Study do not conclude that retinol supplements increased the risk for hip fractures. After adjusting for age, protein, vitamins D and K, calcium, caffeine, and alcohol intakes, BMI, hormone therapy use, smoking, ethnicity, and region of clinical center, the association between vitamin A intake and the risk of fracture was not statistically significant. Only a modest increase in total fracture risk with high vitamin A and retinol intakes (3 times RDA) was observed in the low vitamin D-intake group (11% of RDA) (Caire-Juvera, 2009).

High serum levels of vitamin A can be harmful in pregnant women due to the teratogenic effects on the fetus. Hypervitaminosis A has been reported in 47% of sleeve gastrectomy patients taking 150% of the RDA for vitamin A in the form of retinol (Aarts, 2010).

Based on the research data, vitamin manufacturers have increased the levels of beta-carotenes and decreased the levels of retinol to reduce the risk of potential toxicity.

Signs and symptoms associated with an acute vitamin A toxicity, include nausea, vomiting, anorexia, irritability, drowsiness, altered mental status, abdominal pain, blurred vision, headache and muscle pain with weakness. Signs and symptoms associated with chronic toxicity include anorexia, alopecia, dry mucus membranes, skin erythema, exanthema, cheilitis, pruritus, brittle nails, severe headache, pseudotumor cerebri, insomnia, fatigue, conjunctivitis, unplanned weight loss, changes in bone metabolism by increasing bone resorption, bone fracture, bone and joint pain, anemia, diarrhea, petechiae, epistaxis, hepatosplenomegaly, hyperostosis, ataxia, papilledema and diplopia. Refer to Figure 9.7.-9.9.

Practical Applications for NFPA: Vitamin A

Vitamin A deficiencies and toxicities are unique to patients with certain medical conditions and lifestyle choices. The medical history, in addition to, the dietary intake and supplement use or misuse data will direct you to focus your assessment on physical changes associated with a deficiency or toxicity.

For patients at risk for a vitamin A insufficiency, use NFPA to determine if the clinical findings, dietary intake data and vitamin supplement intake data support a possible vitamin A deficiency. Consider recommending a dark-adaptation threshold (DAT) test. The DAT is a vision test that measures the adjustment of the eye occurring under low levels of illumination and has been correlated with serum vitamin A levels (Carney, 1980).

Laboratory tests to assess for vitamin A deficiency include serum retinol, retinol binding protein, zinc and complete blood count. Nutrition diagnoses that may apply include suboptimal vitamin A intake, excessive alcohol intake, impaired nutrient utilization, altered nutrition-related lab values, limited adherence to nutrition-related recommendations.

For patients at risk for a hypervitaminosis A, use NFPA to determine if the clinical findings, dietary intake data and vitamin supplement use or misuse support a possible vitamin A overload. It is likely that other diagnostic tests will be ordered by the physician to rule out other etiologies. Laboratory tests to assess for vitamin A toxicity include serum retinol, liver function tests, complete blood count. Nutrition diagnoses that may apply include excessive vitamin A intake, altered nutrition-related lab values, limited adherence to nutrition-related recommendations or harmful beliefs about nutrition-related topics (i.e. supplement use).

Vitamin D

Vitamin D is discussed in chapter 8 from the perspective of a insufficiency or deficiency state. As a fat-soluble vitamin, there is a potential for overload. Vitamin D has received considerable media coverage as a 'natural' way to reduce risk for numerous chronic diseases. While the emerging data is promising, some consumers may believe that taking more than the recommended amounts is beneficial.

Vitamin D Toxicity

Vitamin D toxicity is rare because it is nearly impossible to get too much vitamin D from sunlight or from foods with the exception of consuming high volumes of cod liver oil. Nearly all vitamin D overdoses come from supplements. The UL for vitamin D is 4,000 IU/d.

Acute toxicity effects are characteristic of hypercalcemia and may include muscle weakness, apathy, headache, anorexia, irritability, nausea, vomiting, and bone pain. Chronic toxicity effects include the above symptoms and constipation, anorexia, abdominal cramps, polydipsia, polyuria, backache, hyperlipidemia, and hypercalcemia. Proteinuria, urinary casts, azotemia, declining renal status and metastatic calcifications can develop. The long term effects of calcinosis include hypertension and cardiac arrhythmias.

Practical Applications for NFPA: Vitamin D

Vitamin D toxicities are unique to patients with certain lifestyle choices. The medical history, in addition to the dietary intake and supplement use or misuse data will direct you to focus your assessment on physical changes associated with toxicity. For vitamin D deficiencies refer to Chapter 8.

Laboratory tests to assess for vitamin D overload are elevated 25(OH)D (> 150 ng/mL; > 375 nmol/L) and serum calcium > 11 mg/dL. Nutrition diagnoses that may apply include excessive vitamin D intake, altered nutrition-related lab values, limited adherence to nutrition-related recommendations or harmful beliefs about nutrition-related topics (i.e. supplement use).

Vitamin E

Vitamin E is a group of compounds including tocopherols and tocotrienols. Vitamin E was once purported to be an 'anti-aging' vitamin and played a significant role in preventing cardiovascular disease. However, findings in large random controlled studies do not support these theories (Stephens, 1996; Traber, 2008; Yusuf, 2000).

Vitamin E has also been purported to play a role in cancer prevention. However, recent studies suggest that vitamin E raised risk for prostate cancer, and that risk was mitigated by selenium supplementation (Klein, 2011).

Vitamin E Deficiency

Vitamin E deficiency is common in developing countries due to prolonged dietary insufficiency. However, vitamin E deficiency among adults in developed countries is uncommon and often secondary to fat malabsorption. Vitamin deficiencies related to cystic fibrosis, chronic cholestatic liver disease, abetalipoproteinemia, short-bowel syndrome, and other malabsorption syndromes may lead to varying degrees of neurologic deficits.

Vitamin E deficiency causes fragility of erythrocytes resulting in hemolytic anemia and degeneration of neurons. Vitamin E deficiency symptoms progress from hyporeflexia, ataxia, limitation in upward gaze, nyctalopia and profound muscle weakness (Tanyel, 1997). Complete blindness, cardiac arrhythmia, and dementia may occur in patients in whom vitamin E deficiency has been prolonged and severe.

Vitamin E Toxicity

Vitamin E is one of the least toxic lipid soluble vitamins. However, since it is promoted to reduce risk for numerous chronic diseases, the potential for overload exists. Megadoses of vitamin E can antagonize the functions of other fat soluble vitamins (Booth, 2004).

Acute toxicity effects associated with megadoses of vitamin E include nausea, gastric distress, abdominal cramps, diarrhea, headache, fatigue, easy bruising and prolonged prothrombin time and activated partial thromboplastin time, inhibition of platelet aggregation, diplopia (at dosages as low as 300 IU), muscle weakness, and creatinuria. Chronic toxicity effects include all of the above, suppression of other antioxidants, and increased risk of hemorrhagic stroke.

Practical Applications for NFPA: Vitamin E

Vitamin E deficiencies and toxicities are unique to patients with certain medical conditions and lifestyle choices. The medical history, in addition to, the dietary intake data and supplement use or misuse data will direct you to focus your assessment on physical changes associated with a deficiency or toxicity. Diagnosis is based on clinical findings. Laboratory assessment includes measuring the ratio of plasma α-tocopherol to total plasma lipids. A low ratio suggests vitamin E deficiency. Measuring erythrocyte hemolysis in response to peroxide can suggest a vitamin E deficiency, but this test is nonspecific. Hemolysis increases as vitamin E deficiency impairs erythrocyte stability.

For vitamin E deficiency, nutrition diagnoses that may apply include suboptimal vitamin E intake, impaired nutrient utilization, altered nutrition-related lab values, limited adherence to nutrition-related recommendations.

Laboratory assessment for a toxicity include prothrombin time (PT), activated partial thromboplastin time (aPTT) and bleeding times. Nutrition diagnoses that may apply include excessive vitamin E intake, altered nutrition-related lab values, limited adherence to nutrition-related recommendations or harmful beliefs about nutrition-related topics (i.e. supplement use).

Vitamin K

Vitamin K is a lipid-soluble vitamin that plays a role in the production of coagulation proteins, in bone metabolism and inhibition of vascular calcification. Requirements for vitamin K are met through dietary sources (i.e. K1 phylloquinone) and synthesis by colonic bacteria (i.e. K2 menaquinone). Unlike other lipid soluble vitamins, there are minimal body stores of vitamin K. Dietary deprivation can rapidly deplete body stores. The body compensates for varying dietary intake by recycling vitamin K. Anticoagulant medications (i.e. warfarin) reduce the liver's ability to recycle vitamin K.

Vitamin K Deficiency

Vitamin K deficiency is uncommon in healthy adults, but is reported in those with malnutrition, alcoholism and with long term use of TPN. High dose vitamin E supplements can antagonize vitamin K and prolong the prothrombin time.

Adults at risk of vitamin K deficiency include multiple abdominal surgeries, parenchymal liver disease, cystic fibrosis, inflammatory bowel disease, disseminated intravascular coagulation, polycythemia vera, nephrotic syndrome, and leukemia. Malabsorption syndrome affects vitamin K absorption in the ileum. Celiac sprue, tropical sprue, Crohn's disease, ulcerative colitis, *Ascaris* infection, bacterial overgrowth, chronic pancreatitis, and short bowel syndrome resulting from multiple abdominal surgeries can be involved in impaired absorption of vitamin K.

Biliary diseases that cause maldigestion of fat may lead to a deficiency of vitamin K. These include common duct obstruction due to stones and strictures, primary biliary cirrhosis, cholangiocarcinoma, and chronic cholestasis.

Medications that can precipitate a vitamin K deficiency include cephalosporin, warfarin, salicylates, anticonvulsants, and certain sulfa drugs.

Clinical findings suggesting a vitamin K deficiency include ecchymosis, petechiae, hematomas, menorrhagia, hematuria, gum bleeding and oozing of blood at surgical or puncture sites. Laboratory test results associated with a vitamin K deficiency include an elevated serum prothrombin time (PT) and activated partial thromboplastin time (aPTT). However, it is not uncommon for these patients to have an elevated PT level and a normal aPTT level. The most sensitive marker is the high level of des-gamma-carboxy prothrombin (DCP), measured with appropriate antibodies.

Vitamin K Toxicity

Phylloquinone (K1) is not toxic when consumed orally, even in large amounts. However, menadione, a synthetic form of a vitamin K precursor that can be converted to menaquinone can cause toxicity. Large doses of menadione have been reported to cause adverse outcomes including hemolytic anemia due to G6PD deficiency, neonatal brain or liver damage, or neonatal death in some rare cases. In the United States, menadione supplements are banned by the U.S. Food and Drug Administration because of their potential toxicity.

Practical Applications for NFPA: Vitamin K

Vitamin K deficiencies are unique to patients with certain medical conditions and lifestyle choices. The medical history, in addition to, the dietary intake and supplement use or misuse data will direct you to focus your assessment on physical changes associated with a deficiency.

Diagnosis is based on clinical findings. Laboratory assessment for a deficiency includes an elevation in the level of serum PT and aPTT. Nutrition diagnoses that may apply include suboptimal vitamin K intake, impaired nutrient utilization, altered nutrition-related lab values, food-medication interaction, limited adherence to nutrition-related recommendations.

Water-Soluble Vitamins

Water soluble vitamins include thiamin, riboflavin, niacin, vitamin B_6, biotin, vitamin B_{12}, pantothenic acid, folic acid and ascorbic acid. These compounds are soluble in water and excreted in the urine. The body does not store appreciable quantities of the water soluble vitamins.

Thiamin

Thiamin is a water-soluble B vitamin that is absorbed in the jejunum by both an active transport and passive processes. Healthy adults can store up to 30 mg of thiamin in the skeletal muscles. Excess intakes are excreted by the kidney. Thiamin has a half-life of 9-18 days and is essentially nontoxic.

Thiamin Deficiency: Beriberi

Thiamin deficiency is reported in developing countries in which the diet is low in thiamin (i.e. cassava is staple) or high in foods containing thiaminases that decrease absorption (i.e. milled rice, shrimp, mussels, clams, fresh fish, and raw animal tissues). It is rarely reported in healthy adults living in developed countries with food fortification programs.

Adults may become deficient in thiamin either by sub-optimal dietary intakes, high alcohol intake with low nutrient diets or by excessive loss (i.e. prolonged vomiting). Prolonged diarrhea may impair the body's ability to absorb thiamin and severe liver disease impairs its use.

Beriberi is observed in patients on long-term peritoneal dialysis without thiamin replacement, persons undergoing long-term starvation, alcohol abuse, following bariatric surgery or persons receiving intravenous fluids with high glucose concentration. Patients with chronic alcoholism often have low thiamin intake, impaired thiamin uptake and storage, and accelerated destruction of thiamin diphosphate increasing the likelihood of beriberi.

Bariatric beriberi has been reported following Roux-en Y gastric bypass, adjustable gastric band and gastrectomy. The most commonly reported form of beriberi is Wernicke-Korsakoff syndrome. It can occur 2-3 months following bariatric surgery and is associated with protracted vomiting, rapid weight loss and suboptimal thiamin intakes from food and supplements.

Early symptoms of a thiamin deficiency are nonspecific including fatigue and vomiting. As body stores are depleted, neurologic signs and symptoms emerge including horizontal nystagmus, palsies of the eye movements, and pretibial edema. Patients may have difficulty climbing stairs, standing on one leg, ataxia, and bilateral symmetric lower extremity paresthesias with burning pain. Progressive mental impairment leads to confusion, memory impairment, confabulation, delusions, hallucinations or psychosis. The neurological changes in beriberi are similar to those seen in vitamin B12 deficiency.

Cardiovascular symptoms include tachycardia, chest pain, heart failure and hypotension. Gastroenterologic symptoms include anorexia and abdominal discomfort.

Medication-induced folate deficiency can indirectly trigger a thiamin deficiency. Thiamin pyrophosphate serves as a coenzyme in a variety of metabolic processes. In these processes, thiamin pyrophosphate is regenerated via the donation of a proton from the reduced form of nicotinamide adenine dinucleotide (NADH). Folate is essential to having enough dihydrofolate reductase to regenerate NADH from its oxidative form. This regeneration allows NADH to continue to be present to regenerate thiamin pyrophosphate without being consumed in the process. If folate is deficient in cells, thiamin is not be converted to its active form.

Other medications that reduce levels of thiamin in the body include digoxin, furosemide and phenytoin.

Thiamin: Toxicity

Acute toxicity of thiamin is rare, but has been reported in patients on TPN receiving more than 100-fold the recommended intake. Symptoms of a thiamin toxicity include tachycardia, hypotension, cardiac dysrhythmias, headache, anaphylaxis, vasodilation, weakness and convulsions.

Practical Applications for NFPA: Thiamin

Thiamin deficiencies are unique to patients with certain medical conditions and lifestyle choices. The medical history, in addition to, the dietary intake and supplement use data will direct you to focus your assessment on physical changes associated with a deficiency or toxicity.

For practical reasons, replacing thiamin is often the first step in diagnosing a deficiency. If the patient responds to treatment, it is safe to assume that thiamin deficiency was a contributing factor. Other tests may be ordered to rule out other co-morbidities including a vitamin B12 deficiency.

Laboratory assessment of thiamin status is not readily available in many settings. Plasma and serum levels of thiamin reflect recent dietary changes and may be misleading. The most appropriate way to measure thiamin status is to measure thiamin diphosphate in whole blood. Also a pyruvate level of >1 mg/dL is a reliable indicator of deficiency and erythrocyte transketolase activity of <0.017 U/dL indicates deficiency. Nutrition diagnoses that may apply include suboptimal thiamin intake, excessive alcohol intake, impaired nutrient utilization, altered nutrition-related lab values, and limited adherence to nutrition-related recommendations.

Niacin

Niacin is a water soluble B vitamin absorbed in the stomach and small intestine. Dietary tryptophan can be utilized to meet dietary requirements. Megadoses of nicotinic acid are known to reduce serum cholesterol and are commonly prescribed with other lipid-lowering medications.

Niacin: Deficiency

Primary niacin deficiency results from extremely low intake of both niacin and tryptophan, which usually occurs in areas where maize constitutes a substantial part of the diet. Bound niacin, found in maize, is not assimilated in the GI tract unless it has been previously treated with alkali. Corn protein is also deficient in tryptophan. Deficiencies of protein and many B vitamins commonly accompany primary niacin deficiency.

Secondary niacin deficiency may be due to diarrhea, cirrhosis, or alcoholism. Pellagra also may occur in carcinoid syndrome in which tryptophan is diverted to form 5-hydroxytryptophan and serotonin and in Hartnup disease in which absorption of tryptophan by the intestine and kidneys is defective.

The most common symptoms of niacin deficiency involve the skin, digestive system, and the nervous system. The symptoms of pellagra are referred to as the three D's: dermatitis, diarrhea, and dementia. In the skin, a thick, scaly, darkly pigmented rash develops symmetrically in areas exposed to sunlight. Lesions can develop in a glove-like distribution on the hands (pellagrous glove) or in a boot-shaped distribution on the feet and legs (pellagrous boot). Sunlight causes Casal's necklace and butterfly-shaped lesions on the face. GI symptoms in the early stages of a niacin deficiency include burning in the pharynx and esophagus, glossitis, abdominal discomfort with distention and constipation. Later, nausea, vomiting, and diarrhea may occur. Diarrhea is often bloody because of bowel hyperemia and ulceration. Neurologic symptoms include headache, apathy, fatigue, depression, disorientation, memory loss, psychosis and encephalopathy that are characterized by impaired consciousness. If untreated, pellagra is ultimately fatal. Refer to Figures 9.10-9.13.

Niacin: Toxicity

Niacin from foods is not known to cause adverse effects. Pharmacological doses of nicotinic acid include flushing of the skin primarily on the face, arms, and chest, pruritus, nausea and vomiting.

Practical Applications for NFPA: Niacin

Niacin deficiencies and toxicities are rare. Side effects from pharmacological doses of nicotinic acid are managed by changing the dosage or used in combination with other lipid lowering medications. Nutrition diagnoses for a niacin deficiency that may apply include suboptimal niacin intake, impaired nutrient utilization, suboptimal protein intake or limited adherence to nutrition-related recommendations. For niacin toxicity, nutrition diagnoses that may apply include excessive niacin intake, or harmful beliefs about food or nutrition-related topics (supplements).

Folate

Folate is a water soluble B vitamin absorbed in the duodenum and proximal jejunum. Patients may lose up to 100 mcg in urine or feces daily. The liver stores of folate are estimated to be 11-28 mg and are depleted within a few months after malabsorptive surgeries.

Folic acid is the synthetic form of folate that is found in supplements and added to fortified foods. It functions as a coenzyme in numerous reactions that involve DNA synthesis, purine synthesis, generation of methylfolate and amino acid interconversions of several indispensable amino acids (i.e. histidine, serine, glycine, homocysteine to methionine).

Folate Deficiency

Folate deficiency affects the DNA biosynthesis and methylation cycles. The effect on the DNA biosynthesis cycle reduces cell division. It is manifest in the rapidly dividing cells of the bone marrow, and results in anemia, neutropenia, and thrombocytopenia. In the gastric mucosal cells the reduction in cell division leads to inflammatory changes. Reduction in the methylation cycle results in elevated homocysteine, a biomarker of folate deficiency, is also associated with hypercoagulability and cardiovascular disease.

A folate deficiency can occur when needs increase, there is suboptimal intake from foods or supplements and when folate loss increases. Medical conditions that increase the need for folate include pregnancy and lactation. Increased loss of folate is seen in patients undergoing chronic dialysis, chronic hemolytic disease, exfoliative dermatitis, liver disease and alcohol abuse. Intestinal malabsorption of folate occurs in disorders of the small intestine, such as tropical sprue, celiac disease, after extensive intestinal resection and following weight loss surgery.

Gehrer (2010) found 22% post-op sleeve gastrectomy patients have insufficient levels of folate. Folate stores can be depleted within a few months post-op unless replenished by dietary sources and supplements. Symptoms of a early stage folate deficiency include fatigue, weakness, headaches, impaired concentration, palpitations, diarrhea, sore red tongue with a smooth shiny surface, and yellow tinged pallor. However laboratory test results for hemoglobin, hematocrit and MCV are within normal ranges. In severe stage disease, patients present with pancytopenia, symptomatic megaloblastic anemia, elevated MCV and ferritin with low hemoglobin, serum iron and hematocrit. Diagnosis is confirmed by the presence of low serum folate, low erythrocyte folate and elevated plasma homocysteine. Cobalamin deficiency must be ruled out before initiating folic acid therapy, as the therapy may mask a deficiency and aggravate neurologic manifestations of an underlying vitamin B12 deficiency. A normal methylmalonic acid (MMA) level will differentiate folate deficiency from vitamin B12 deficiency because MMA levels rise in vitamin B12 deficiency but not in folate deficiency.

Medications that interfere with the metabolism of folate may also increase the need for folate and the risk of deficiency. Folate antagonists include dilantin, phenytoin, primidone, metformin, sulfasalazine, triamterene, methotrexate and barbiturates. Alcohol interferes with the absorption of folate and increases the amount excreted. In addition, many alcoholics have poor quality diets that contain suboptimal amounts of folate (Cravo, 1996; Gloria, 1997).

Folate Toxicity
Folate intake from food is not associated with any health risk. The risk of toxicity from folic acid intake from multivitamins and/or fortified foods is low because body stores of folate are limited. However, concerns regarding safety are limited to higher dose synthetic folic acid intake.

High doses folic acid can mask a vitamin B12 deficiency by resolving the pernicious anemia, but not correcting the neurological damage that occurs with a vitamin B12 deficiency.

The role of folate supplements in cancer risk is controversial. While dietary folate may be protective against colorectal cancer, high doses of supplemental folic acid may actually accelerate tumor growth in cancer patients. A recent chemopreventive trial in patients with a history of colorectal adenoma found a positive assoication between supplementation of 1 mg/day of folic acid with advanced colorectal lesions as well as increased risk (>2-fold) for the presence of three or more colorectal adenomas (Cole, 2007). However, other trials have not found evidence that folic acid supplementation increases risk of colorectal adenoma recurrence (Wu, 2009; Figueiredo, 2009; Logan, 2008).

Two other trials found folic acid supplementation to be associated with increased risk of prostate cancer (Cole, 2007, Logan, 2008). A recent meta-analysis of seven randomized controlled trials found that supplemental folic acid use (800 mcg-40 mg/day [median 2.5 mg/day] for 2.0-7.3 years) did not increase risk for overall cancer incidence or cancer-related mortality (Clarke, 2010). Human observational studies as well as animal studies on high-dose folic acid supplements and cancer have reported mixed results. More research is needed to determine the role of high-dose folic acid supplements in cancer progression.

Practical Applications for NFPA: Folate
Folate intake from food is not associated with adverse effects. The role of folic acid in fortified foods and in dietary supplements remains controversial. NFPA is a useful tool

for identifying signs of megaloblastic anemia in conjunction with laboratory tests results, medications and dietary intake. Nutrition diagnoses for a folate deficiency that may apply include suboptimal folate intake, impaired nutrient utilization, altered nutrition-related lab values, food-medication interaction, altered GI function or limited adherence to nutrition-related recommendations.

The toxic effects of megadoses of folate are not as evident and may entail subtle long term effects. For folate toxicity, nutrition diagnoses that may apply include excessive folate intake, or harmful beliefs about food or nutrition-related topics (supplements).

Vitamin B$_6$

Vitamin B$_6$ is a water soluble vitamin that includes a group of closely related compounds: pyridoxine, pyridoxal, and pyridoxamine. Vitamin B$_6$ is present in most foods and dietary deficiencies are rare. However, even though it is a water soluble vitamin, megadoses have resulted in overload with lingering side effects.

Vitamin B$_6$ Deficiency

Secondary deficiency of vitamin B$_6$ may result from malnutrition, malabsorption, alcoholism, use of pyridoxine-inactivating drugs (e.g. anticonvulsants, isoniazid). Symptoms can include peripheral neuropathy, anemia, depression, confusion, EEG abnormalities, and seizures. Deficiency causes a pellagra-like syndrome with seborrheic dermatitis, glossitis, and cheilosis.

Vitamin B$_6$ Toxicity

The ingestion of megadoses (> 500 mg/day) of pyridoxine has been purported to treat carpal tunnel syndrome and premenstrual syndrome. The efficacy of this regimen is unproved. It may cause peripheral neuropathy with deficits in a stocking-glove distribution, including progressive sensory ataxia and severe impairment of position and vibration senses. Senses of touch, temperature, and pain are less affected. Motor and central nervous systems are usually intact. After vitamin B_6 supplements are discontinued, recovery is slow and, for some patients, incomplete.

Practical Applications for NFPA: Vitamin B_6

Diagnosis of vitamin B_6 deficiency or toxicity is usually based on clinical findings and laboratory test results. Fasting pyridoxal 5'-phosphate blood test accurately indicates vitamin B_6 nutrition status.

Nutrition diagnoses for a vitamin B_6 deficiency that may apply include suboptimal vitamin B_6 intake, impaired nutrient utilization or altered nutriton-related lab values. limited adherence to nutrition-related recommendations, or harmful beliefs about food or nutrition-related topics (supplements). For vitamin B_6 toxicity, nutrition diagnoses that may apply include excessive vitamin B_6 intake, or harmful beliefs about food or nutrition-related topics (supplements).

Vitamin B_{12}

Vitamin B12 is a water-soluble vitamin that exists in several forms and contains the mineral cobalt. Methylcobalamin and 5-deoxyadenosylcobalamin are the forms of vitamin B12 that are active in human metabolism. The form of cobalamin used in most supplements, cyanocobalamin. It is readily converted to 5-deoxyadenosyl and methylcobalamin in the body. Vitamin B12 is required for proper red blood cell formation, neurological function, and DNA synthesis.

Vitamin B12 is present in meat, poultry, seafood, and to a lesser extent milk. It is not generally present in plant products or yeast. Absorption of dietary sources of vitamin B12 require sufficient hydrochloric acid and gastric protease in the stomach to cleave the protein carrier. When synthetic vitamin B12 is added to fortified foods and dietary supplements, it is already in free form. Free vitamin B12 then combines with intrinsic factor (IF), a glycoprotein secreted by the stomach's parietal cells. The B12- IF complex binds to mucosal cells in the ileum and B12 is absorbed. When vitamin B12 is released from the mucosal cell, it binds to transport proteins in the bloodstream and goes to the bone marrow for use in the liver or other tissues.

In healthy adults, body stores of cobalamin usually exceed 1000 mcg and the daily requirement is about 1 mcg. Strict adherence to a vegetarian diet for more than 5 years usually is required to deplete body stores.

Vitamin B$_{12}$ Deficiency

The most common causes of vitamin B12 deficiency are pernicious anemia, food-bound vitamin B12 malabsorption and suboptimal dietary intake. Pernicious anemia and vitamin B12 malabsorption become more common with increasing age. Other etiologies include malabsorptive surgical procedures, bacterial overgrowth in which the bacteria compete with the body for cobalamin and insufficient pancreatic protease (e.g., chronic pancreatitis, Zollinger-Ellison syndrome).

Pernicious anemia is a chronic illness caused by impaired absorption of vitamin B12 because of a lack of intrinsic factor (IF) in gastric secretions. It is associated with gastric atrophy that leads to the destruction of parietal cells, achlorhydria, and failure to produce intrinsic factor, resulting in vitamin B12 malabsorption.

Pernicious anemia probably is an autoimmune disorder with a genetic predisposition. It is more common than expected in families of patients with pernicious anemia. Antiparietal cell antibodies occur in 90% of patients with pernicious anemia but in only 5% of healthy adults. If pernicious anemia is left untreated, it causes vitamin B12 deficiency, leading to anemia and neurological disorders, even in the presence of adequate dietary intake of vitamin B12.

Individuals who have had Roux-en-Y gastric by-pass (RYGB) and sleeve gastrectomy (SG), have both incomplete digestion and release of vitamin B12 from foods. The surgical procedure impairs the effectiveness of parietal cells to produce IF and reduces the production of hydrochloric acid in the stomach. Hypochlorhydria results in a reduced ability to cleave dietary vitamin B12 from its protein carrier. IF is required for intestinal absorption of vitamin B12. Individuals who have had a bowel resection or disease of the terminal ileum will also have impaired vitamin B12 utilization due to insufficient absorptive surfaces (Aills, 2008; Hakeam, 2009; Himpens, 2006).

Signs and symptoms of vitamin B12 deficiency are insidious and vague. The classic triad of weakness, sore tongue, and paresthesias may not be recognized by the patient as signs of a vitamin deficiency. Anorexia is common and about 50% of patients will have unplanned weight loss. Other physical signs and symptoms include lemon-yellow waxy pallor with premature whitening of the hair, loss of sense of touch, stiffness in arms and legs, and tachycardia (Bickley, 2009). Refer to Figure 5.15.

A sore, smooth, beefy red tongue with loss of papillae is reported in approximately 50% of patients. Occasionally, red patches are observed on the edges of the dorsum of the tongue. Patients may report burning or soreness on the anterior third of the tongue. These symptoms may be associated with changes in taste and loss of appetite. Constipation or diarrhea are common complaints. These symptoms have been attributed to megaloblastic changes of the cells of the intestinal mucosa.

Neurologic symptoms are paresthesias, weakness, clumsiness, and an unsteady gait. Ask the patient if he/she feels more unsteady or clumsy in a dark room. These symptoms become worse in a dark room because they reflect the loss of proprioception in a patient who is unable to rely upon vision for compensation. These neurologic symptoms are due to myelin degeneration and loss of nerve fibers in the dorsal and lateral columns of the spinal cord and cerebral cortex. Memory loss, irritability, and personality changes are common. Megaloblastic madness is less common and can be manifested by delusions, hallucinations, outbursts, and paranoid schizophrenic ideation.

Medications that reduce the absorption of vitamin B12 include omeprazole, lansoprazole, Tagamet, Pepcid, Zantac, cholestyramine, chloramphenicol, neomycin, colchicine, and metformin.

Biomarkers of a vitamin B12 deficiency include low levels of hemoglobin, hematocrit, erythrocyte counts, lymphocyte and platelet counts, reticulocyte count and serum vitamin B12. The indirect bilirubin level may be elevated because pernicious anemia is a hemolytic disorder associated with increased turnover of bilirubin. In addition, serum iron, MCV, ferritin, methylmalonic acid, homocysteine, lactic dehydrogenase and antiparietal cell antibodies levels are elevated (Litchford, 2011).

Vitamin B$_{12}$ Toxicity

No toxic or adverse effects have been associated with large intakes of vitamin B12 from food or supplements in healthy adults. Doses as high as 1 mg (1000 mcg) daily by mouth or 1 mg monthly by intramuscular injection have been used to treat pernicious anemia without significant side effects. When high doses of vitamin B12 are given orally, only a small percentage can be absorbed.

Practical Applications for NFPA: Vitamin B$_{12}$

Vitamin B12 deficiency is easily overlooked because the early signs are insidious and ambiguous. Vegans need supplemental vitamin B12 to meet their requirements. Also, individuals over the age of 50 should obtain their vitamin B12 in supplements or fortified foods because of the increased likelihood of food-bound vitamin B12 malabsorption. In older adults, falls and subsequent fractures may be due to neurological symptoms of an unrecognized vitamin B12 deficiency. Nutrition diagnoses that may apply include suboptimal vitamin B12 intake, suboptimal protein intake, impaired nutrient utilization, altered nutrition-related lab values, food-medication interaction, limited adherence to nutrition-related recommendations, or harmful beliefs about food or nutrition-related topics.

Biotin

Biotin is a water soluble B vitamin. The dietary requirements are met through foods, intestinal synthesis and recycling biotin. Biotin deficiency rarely occurs in healthy adults who consume a variety of foods unless they are being treated either with certain anticonvulsants or with broad-spectrum antibiotics. The toxicity of biotin appears to be very low and only reported in animal models.

Biotin Deficiency
Biotin deficiency has been demonstrated in prolonged parenteral feeding without biotin supplementation and with consumption of raw egg white for a many weeks to years. Avidin is an antimicrobial protein found in egg white that binds biotin and prevents its absorption. Cooking egg white denatures avidin, rendering it susceptible to digestion and therefore unable to prevent the absorption of dietary biotin.

Clinical manifestations of a biotin deficiency are confined to the intestinal tract, skin, hair, central nervous system, and peripheral nervous system. The first signs that develop in a deficiency state are associated with the skin and hair. Dry skin is common and is often associated with severe seborrheic dermatitis. The skin lesions provide an ideal environment for fungal infections that may be resistant to treatment until the biotin-deficient state is reversed. The hair quickly becomes fine and brittle, and total alopecia often develops. As the deficiency progresses neurological findings present initially with mild depression, which may progress to profound lassitude to somnolence. Myalgias, hyperesthesias and paresthesias are common findings. Intestinal tract symptoms also develop such as nausea, vomiting and anorexia.

Prolonged use of phenytoin, primidone, and carbamazepine, inhibit biotin transport across the intestinal mucosa and may lead to biotin deficiency. Evidence suggests that these anticonvulsants accelerate biotin catabolism.

Hair loss after bariatric surgery often occurs between the third and sixth month after surgery and can last 6 to 12 months or more. Biotin supplementation is a common intervention although there is no consensus on treatment (Bruginsky, 2001).

Practical Applications for NFPA: Biotin
The diagnosis of biotin deficiency is primarily based on clinical findings and dietary intake data (i.e. raw egg whites). Nutrition diagnoses that may apply include suboptimal biotin intake, impaired nutrient utilization, limited adherence to nutrition-related recommendations, or undesirable food choices.

Iodine
Iodine is an essential element that enables the thyroid gland to produce thyroid hormones. The thyroid is a butterfly-shaped gland that lies in front of the trachea, just below the larynx. It is unique among endocrine glands because it has a large store of hormones and a slow rate of turnover. Thyroxine (T4) and triiodothyronine (T3) are produced by the thyroid gland when the anterior pituitary gland releases thyroid-stimulating hormone (TSH). Iodine is required to form T4.

Iodine Deficiency: Goiter
A 'goiter' is an abnormal enlargement of the thyroid gland and its presence does not necessarily mean that the thyroid gland is malfunctioning. A goiter can occur in a gland that is producing too much hormone (hyperthyroidism), too little hormone (hypothyroidism), or the correct amount of hormone (euthyroidism). A goiter indicates there is a

condition present which is causing the thyroid to grow abnormally.

One of the most common causes of goiter formation is iodine deficiency, although it is rarely seen in the United States. The primary activity of the thyroid gland is to concentrate iodine from the blood to make thyroid hormone. Sub-optimal levels of iodine in the blood equates to insufficient production of thyroid hormone. To counteract the hypothyroid state, thyroid stimulating hormone (TSH) is released which stimulates the thyroid to produce thyroid hormone and to grow in size. In hyperthyroidism, the pituitary senses too much thyroid hormone and it stops secreting TSH. In spite of this, the thyroid gland continues to grow and make thyroid hormone. Blood tests for T3, T4, TSH and the presence of thyroid autoantibodies are primarily used for diagnosis. Refer to Table 9.1 for signs and symptoms of thyroid dysfunction and Figures 9.14.-9.17. Graves' disease is the most common form of hyperthyroidism. It is an autoimmune condition in which the body produces antibodies that destroy the thyroid-stimulating hormone (TSH) receptor. As a result, the thyroid gland is inappropriately stimulated with ensuing gland enlargement and increasing thyroid hormone production. Other classic hallmarks include exophthalmos (marked prominence of eyeball), and pretibial myxedema (localized lesions of the skin resulting from the deposition of hyaluronic acid).

Hashimoto's thyroiditis is the most common cause of hypothyroidism in the United States. It is an autoimmune condition in which the body produces antibodies that destroy the cells of the thyroid gland. While goiter is common, it is not always seen in Hashimoto's thyroiditis.

Untreated hyperthyroidism can lead to atrial fibrillation, congestive heart failure, osteoporosis, arterial thromboembolism, hypertension and neuropsychiatric problems. Untreated hypothyroidism may lead to depression, mental and behavioral impairment, myxedema, hypothermia, hypertension, congestive heart failure, and dyslipidemias.

Table 9.1. Signs and Symptoms of Thyroid Dysfunction

Hyperthyroidism	Hypothyroidism
Fatigue, muscle weakness,	Fatigue, sluggish, forgetful
Tremors	Puffy face & eyelids
Weight loss or gain	Weight gain, difficulty losing weight
Changes in appetite	Constipation
Hair thinning & loss	Hair loss & brittle nails
Heat intolerance	Cold intolerance
Mental slowing, depression	Depression
Insomnia	Hoarse voice
Bulging eyes, starriness of eyes	Pain, stiffness, swelling in joints
Goiter	Goiter
Bradycardia (heart rate < 60 beats/min)	Heart palpitations, tachycardia
Edema	Pale, dry skin
Tense, restless, anxious	Nervousness
	Elevated cholesterol and triglyceride

Zinc

Zinc is an essential trace mineral that plays a role in cell replication, protein synthesis, collagen synthesis, taste, smell and immune function. A daily intake of zinc is required to maintain a steady state because the body has no specialized zinc storage system (Rink, 2000). Zinc is naturally present in some foods, added to others, and available as a dietary supplement. It is also found in many cold lozenges and some over-the-counter medications sold as cold remedies.

Zinc Deficiency

Zinc deficiency may have genetic, nutritional, or metabolic etiologies. Acrodermatitis enteropathica is an autosomal-recessive disease causing severe zinc deficiency through impaired absorption. Acquired zinc deficiency may result from suboptimal nutritional intake, ingestion of foods or drugs that reduce zinc absorption, chronic illness, increased losses of zinc from the body, or increased requirements for zinc. The bioavailability of zinc from vegan diets is lower than from a mixed foods diet. Vegetarians typically eat high levels of legumes and whole grains, which contain phytates that bind zinc and inhibit its absorption. In addition, meat may enhance zinc absorption (Hunt, 2003).

Acquired zinc deficiency is common in developing regions due to malnutrition. In developed regions zinc deficiency is associated with aging and many chronic diseases. As zinc deficiency can present in many ways, it should be considered in patients with at-risk conditions. Conditions that place patients at risk for zinc deficiency include advanced age, celiac disease, Crohn's disease, short bowel syndrome, AIDS enteropathy, ileostomy, chronic diarrhea, enteric fistula output, chronic liver disease, cirrhosis, nephrotic syndrome, diabetes, alcoholism, trauma, burns, and sickle cells anemia. High alcohol consumption was shown to decrease intestinal absorption of zinc and increase urinary zinc excretion (Prasad, 2004).

Losses of zinc occur with large skin wounds, from diarrhea and in urine following trauma or closed head injury. Zinc deficiencies have been reported in 34% of patients following sleeve gastrectomy (Gehrer, 2010). Zinc deficiency in older people contributes to susceptibility to infection and osteoporosis (Haase, 2004).

Medications that promote increased losses of zinc include penicillamine, diuretics, diethylenetriamine pentaacetate and valproate. Calcium supplements should not be taken at the same time as zinc supplements because high levels of calcium interfere with the absorption of zinc (Wood, 1997).

Zinc deficiency is characterized by growth retardation, loss of appetite, and impaired immune function. In more severe cases, it causes impaired glucose tolerance, diarrhea, alopecia, stomatitis, acrodermatitis enteropathica, paronychia, nystagmus, night blindness, blepharitis, delayed sexual maturation, impotence, and hypogonadism in males (IOM, 2001; Prasad, 2004; Wang, 2005; Maret, 2006). Weight loss, delayed healing of wounds (Scholl, 2001; Pories, 1967; Norris 1971; Haggard, 1999), taste abnormalities, and impaired concentration can also occur (King, 2005; Krasovec, 1996; Ploysangam, 1997; Nsihi, 1996, IOM, 2001).

Many of these symptoms are non-specific and often associated with other health conditions. NFPA as part of the nutrition assessment process may be helpful in identifying whether a zinc deficiency is present. Zinc deficiency is difficult to measure adequately using laboratory tests due to its distribution throughout the body as a component of various proteins and nucleic acids (Hunt, 2003; Hambidge, 2007). Plasma or serum zinc levels reflect recent intakes rather than stores (Litchford, 2010) and do not necessarily reflect cellular zinc status due to tight homeostatic control mechanisms (Maret, 2006). Clinical effects of zinc deficiency can be present in the absence of abnormal laboratory indices (Maret, 2006). Other lab tests usually ordered with a suspected zinc deficiency include serum iron, 25(OH)D, folate and vitamin B12.

Zinc Toxicity

Megadoses of zinc have been purported to improve immune function, heal wounds, treat age-related macular degeneration (AMD) and vision loss. Acute adverse effects of high zinc intake include nausea, vomiting, loss of appetite, abdominal cramps, diarrhea, and headaches (IOM, 2001). Intakes of 150–450 mg of zinc per day have been associated with such chronic effects as low copper status, altered iron function, anemia that does not respond to iron or vitamin B12, reduced immune function, and reduced levels of high-density lipoproteins (Hooper, 1980). High zinc intakes can inhibit copper absorption, sometimes producing copper deficiency and associated anemia. Reductions in ceruloplasmin levels have been reported with even moderately high zinc intakes of approximately 60 mg/day for up to 10 weeks (IOM, 2001).

Participants in the Age-Related Eye Disease Study (AREDS, 2001) took 80 mg zinc/d for more than 6 years. Zinc supplementation alone significantly reduced the risk of developing advanced AMD in subjects at higher risk but not in the total study population. Visual acuity loss was not significantly affected by zinc supplementation alone.

Practical Applications for NFPA: Zinc
The diagnosis of a zinc deficiency is primarily based on clinical signs and symptoms of at risk patients and dietary intake data. Nutrition diagnoses that may apply include suboptimal zinc intake, impaired nutrient utilization, limited adherence to nutrition-related recommendations, or excessive alcohol intake.

The diagnosis of a zinc toxicity is primarily based on clinical signs and symptoms of patients taking megadoes of zinc. Nutrition diagnoses that may apply include excessive zinc intake, impaired nutrient utilization or limited adherence to nutrition-related recommendations.

Clinical Nutrition Pearls: HEENT & Nutrition-Related Conditions
The RDN is the member of the healthcare team who is most likely to correlate NFPA findings with nutrient deficiencies or toxicities. Deficiencies are rarely seen in developed countries and easily overlooked or misdiagnosed. Demonstrate your ability to make clinical connections between physical findings, patient symptoms and dietary intake.

Some patients require vitamin mineral supplementation. Recent studies have linked a number of individual vitamins and mineral to a slight increased risk of mortality. The studies were not designed to identify the specific cause of increased mortality. However the authors note that most compounds are toxic at high amounts and long term use might predispose a patient to detrimental outcomes (Mursu, 2011).

Figures 9.1.- 9.4. illustrate NFPA findings in vitamin A deficiency.

Figure 9.1. Follicular hyperkeratosis **Figure 9.2.** Brittle Nails

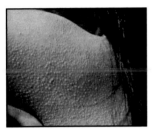 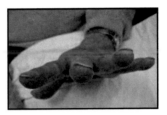

Figure 9.3. Keratomalacia **Figures 9.4.-9.5.** Bitot's Spots

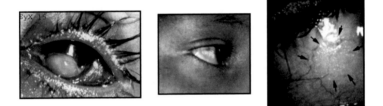

Figures 9.6.- 9.7 illustrate NFPA findings in vitamin A toxicity.

Figure 9.6. Hypercarotenemia   **Figure 9.7.** Petechiae

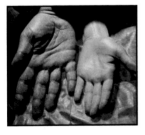 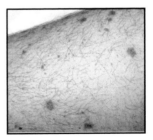

Figures 9.8.-9.9 pretibial myxedema
(thiamin deficiency or hyperthyroidism)

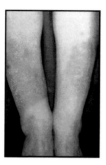 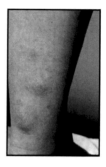

Figures 9.10.-9.11. Pellagra, Casal's necklace
(niacin deficiency)

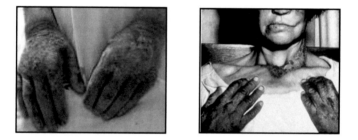

Figures 9.12 -9.13. Megaloblastic Anemia, Glossitis
(folate and B12 deficiencies)

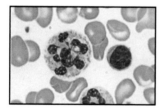 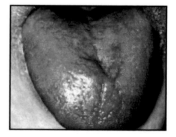

Figures 9.14.- 9.17. illustrate NFPA findings in thyroid dysfunction and iodine imbalance.

Figures 9.14-9.15. Hypothyroidism Before and After Treatment

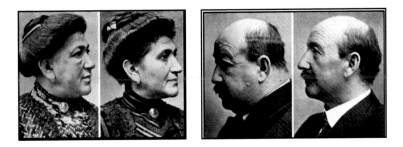

Figures 9.16-9.17. Goiter, Hyperthyroidism: Bulging Eyes

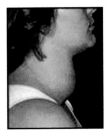
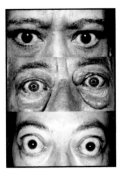

Figures 9.18.-9.19. Blepharitis, Acrodermatitis Enteropathica (zinc deficiency)

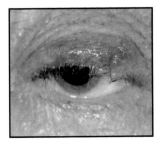
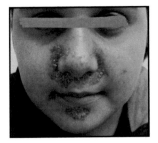

NFPA: Putting the Pieces Together

Mastering NFPA takes time and clinical experience. If you are new to NFPA, identify one or two specific areas in your clinical practice to begin incorporating this tool into your assessments. There are numerous training videos available for free on the Internet. Ask for training at your healthcare facility from the departments of nursing or medicine. Other healthcare team members will be happy to assist you. Shadow another RDN who is using NFPA.

Once you have completed didactic and 'hands on' training, demonstrate your skills and document your competency following the policies of your employer. Use your Professional Development Portfolio to maintain a record of your training. Keep abreast of updates on the characteristics of malnutrition and commit yourself to lifelong learning!

References

Aarts, EO The Gastric Sleeve: Losing Weight as Fast as Micronutrients? OBES SURG, DOI 10.1007/s11695-010-0316-7, Nov 2010.

Aasheim ET, Bjorkman S, Sovik TT, et al. Vitamin status after bariatric surgery: a randomized study of gastric bypass and duodenal switch. Am J Clin Nutr. Jul 2009;90(1):15-22.

Aasheim ET. Night blindness after duodenal switch. Surg Obes Relat Dis. 2008;4(5):685-6

Aasheim ET. Vitamin status after bariatric surgery: a randomized study of gastric bypass and duodenal switch. Am J Clin Nutr 2009;1;15 -22.

Aasheim ET. Wernicke encephalopathy after bariatric surgery. A systematic review. Ann Surg. 2005;248(5):714–20

Aasheim, Erlend T. (2008) Peripheral Neuropathy and Severe Malnutrition following Duodenal Switch. Obesity Surgery 2008 Dec;18(12):1640-3. Epub 2008 May 8.

Abu-Hijleh, G & Padmanabhan, R. Retinoic acid-induced abnormal development of hindlimb joints in the mouse. Eur J Morphol 1997;35:327–36.

Age-Related Eye Disease Study Research Group. A randomized, placebo-controlled, clinical trial of high-dose supplementation with vitamins C and E, beta carotene, and zinc for age-related macular degeneration and vision loss: AREDS report no. 8. Arch Ophthalmol 2001;119:1417-36.

Aills L. Bariatric nutrition guidelines for the surgical weight loss patient. Surg Obes Relat Dis. 2008. Suppl;4(45).

Angstadt JD, Bodziner RA. Peripheral polyneuropathy from thiamine deficiency following laparoscopic Roux-en-Y gastric bypass. Obes Surg. Jun-Jul 2005;15(6):890-2.

Bendich, A & Langseth, L. Safety of vitamin A. AJCN 1989;49:358–71.

Booth, SL Effect of vitamin E supplementation on vitamin K status in adults with normal coagulation status (2004) AJCN 80, 143-148.

Bruginsky A. Biotin supplementation as a treatment for alopecia post gastroplasty. [Monograph]. Sao Paulo: Brazilian Institute of Homeopathic Studies. Specialization in Orthomolecular Nutrition and longevity. São Paulo, 2001:38.

Caire-Juvera, G, Ritenbaugh , C (2008)Vitamin A and retinol intakes and the risk of fractures among participants of the Women's Health Initiative Observational Study. Am J Clin Nutr. 2009 Jan;89(1):323-30.

Cappola AR, Fried LP. Thyroid status, cardiovascular risk, and mortality in older adults. JAMA. Mar 1 2006;295(9):1033-41.

Carney, E. Correlation of Dark Adaptation Test Results with Serum Vitamin A Levels in Diseased Adults J Nutr. 110: 552-557, 1980.

Clarke R, Halsey J, Lewington S, et al. Effects of lowering homocysteine levels with B vitamins on cardiovascular disease, cancer, and cause-specific mortality: Meta-analysis of 8 randomized trials involving 37 485 individuals. Arch Intern Med. 2010;170(18):1622-1631.

Cole BF, Baron JA, Sandler RS, et al. Folic acid for the prevention of colorectal adenomas: a randomized clinical trial. JAMA. 2007;297(21):2351-2359.

Cravo ML, Gloria LM, Selhub J, Nadeau MR, Camilo ME, Hyperhomocysteinemia in chronic alcoholism: Correlation with folate, vitamin B-12, and vitamin B-6 status. Am J Clin Nutr 1996;63:220-4.

DiGiovanna, JJ, Sollitto, RB. Osteoporosis is a toxic effect of long-term etretinate therapy. Arch Dermatol 1995;131:1263–7.

Dolan K, Hatzifotis M, Newbury L, et al. A clinical and nutritional comparison of biliopancreatic diversion with and without duodenal switch. Ann Surg 2004;240:51– 6.

Figueiredo JC, Grau MV, Haile RW, et al. Folic acid and risk of prostate cancer: results from a randomized clinical trial. J Natl Cancer Inst. 2009;101(6):432-435.

Frame, B, Jackson, CE, Reynolds, WA & Umphrey, JE. Hypercalcemia and skeletal effects in chronic hypervitaminosis A. Ann Intern Med 1974;80:44–8.

Gehrer, S Fewer nutrient deficiencies after laparoscopic sleeve gastrectomy than after laparoscopic RNY. Obes Surg. 2010; 20(4):447-53.

Glauser J, Strange GR. Hypothyroidism and hyperthyroidism in the elderly. Emerg Med Rep. 2002;1(2):1-12.

Gloria L, Cravo M, Camilo ME, Resende M, Cardoso JN, Oliveira AG, Leitao CN, Mira FC. Nutritional deficiencies in chronic alcoholics: Relation to dietary intake and alcohol consumption. Am J Gastroenterol 1997;92:485-9.

Gollobin C. Bariatric beriber. Am J Med 2004;117:804-5.

Gollobin C. Bariatric beriberi. Obes Surg. 2002;12:309–311.

Gorstein JL, Dary O. Feasibility of using retinol-binding protein from capillary blood specimens to estimate serum retinol concentrations and the prevalence of vitamin A deficiency in low-resource settings. Public Health Nutr. May 2008;11(5):513-20.

Haase H, Mocchegiani E, Rink L. Correlation between zinc status and immune function in the elderly. Biogerontology. 2006;7:421-428.

Hakeam HA, O'Regan PJ. Impact of laparoscopic sleeve gastrectomy on iron indices: 1 year follow-up. Obes Surg. 2009 (11):1491-6.

Hambidge KM, Krebs NF. Zinc deficiency: a special challenge. J Nutr 2007;137:1101-5.

Hambidge KM, Mild zinc deficiency in human subjects. In: Mills CF, ed. Zinc in Human Biology. New York, NY: Springer-Verlag, 1989:281-96.

Hathcock, JN, Hattan, DG, Jenkins, MY, McDonald, JT, Sundaresan, PR & Wilkening, VL. Evaluation of vitamin A toxicity. Am J Clin Nutr 1990;52:183–202.

Heyneman CA. Zinc deficiency and taste disorders. Ann Pharmacother 1996;30:186-7.

Himpens. A prospective randomized study between laparoscopic gastric banding and laparoscopic isolated sleeve gastrectomy: results after 1 and 3 years . Obesity surgery, 2006. 16 (11),1450 -1456

Hooper PL, Visconti L, Garry PJ, Johnson GE. Zinc lowers high-density lipoprotein-cholesterol levels. J Am Med Assoc 1980;244:1960-1.

Hunt JR. Bioavailability of iron, zinc, and other trace minerals from vegetarian diets. Am J Clin Nutr 2003;78 (3 Suppl):633S-9S.

IOM, FNB. Dietary Reference Intakes for Vitamin A, Vitamin K, Arsenic, Boron, Chromium, Copper, Iodine, Iron, Manganese, Molybdenum, Nickel, Silicon, Vanadium, and Zinc. Washington, DC: National Academy Press, 2001.

Jimenez C, Leets I. A single dose of vitamin A improves haemoglobin concentration, retinol status and phagocytic function of neutrophils in preschool children. Br J Nutr. Dec 15 2009;1-5.

Johnson AR, Munoz A, Gottlieb JL, Jarrard DF. High dose zinc increases hospital admissions due to genitourinary complications. J Urol 2007;177:639-43.

Juhasz-Pocsine K. Neurological complications of gastric bypass surgery for morbid obesity. Neurology. 2007;68:1843–1850.

Kang YJ, Zhou Z. Zinc prevention and treatment of alcoholic liver disease. Mol Aspects Med 2005;26:391-404.

Kindmark, A, Rollman, O, Mallmin, H, Petren-Mallmin, M, Oral isotretinoin therapy in severe acne induces transient suppression of biochemical markers of bone turnover and calcium homeostasis. Acta Derm Venereol 1998;78:266–9.

King JC, Cousins RJ. Zinc. In: Shils ME, Shike M, Ross AC, Caballero B, Cousins, RJ, eds. Modern Nutrition in Health and Disease, 10th ed. Baltimore, MD: Lippincott Williams & Wilkins, 2005:271-85.

Klein EA et al. Vitamin E and the risk of prostate cancer: The Selenium and Vitamin E Cancer Prevention Trial (SELECT). JAMA 2011 Oct 12; 306:1549.

Koffman BM, et al. Neurologic complications after surgery for obesity.Muscle Nerve 2006;33:166-76.

Koike H, Iijima M, Mori K, et al. Postgastrectomy polyneuropathy with thiamine deficiency is identical to beriberi neuropathy. Nutrition. Nov-Dec 2004;20(11-12):961-6.

Krasovec M, Frenk E. Acrodermatitis enteropathica secondary to Crohn's disease. Dermatology 1996;193:361-3.

Logan RF, Grainge MJ, Shepherd VC, Armitage NC, Muir KR. Aspirin and folic acid for the prevention of recurrent colorectal adenomas. Gastroenterology. 2008;134(1):29-38.

Madan AK, Orth WS, Tichansky DS, Ternovits CA. Vitamin and trace mineral levels after laparoscopic gastric bypass. Obes Surg 2006;16:603– 6.

Makarewicz, W Wernicke's syndrome after sleeve gastroectomy. Obes Surg 2007;17(5);704-6.

Maret W, Sandstead HH. Zinc requirements and the risks and benefits of zinc supplementation. J Trace Elem Med Biol 2006;20:3-18.

Matrana MR, Vasireddy S, Davis WE.The skinny on a growing problem: dry beri beri after bariatric surgery. Ann Intern Med. 2008 Dec 2;149(11):842-4.

Munoz EC, Rosado JL, Lopez P, et al. Iron and zinc supplementation improves indicators of vitamin A status of Mexican preschoolers. Am J Clin Nutr. Mar 2000;71(3):789-94.

Mursa, J Dietary supplements and mortality rate in older women. Arch Intern Med. 2011;171(18):1625-1633.

Nautiyal A, et al. Wernicke encephalopathy-an emerging trend after bariatric surgery. Am J Med 2004;117:804-5.

Nishi Y. Zinc and growth. J Am Coll Nutr 1996;15:340-4.

Okada, N, Nomura, M, Morimoto, S, Ogihara, T & Yoshikawa, K. Bone mineral density of the lumbar spine in psoriatic patients with long term etretinate therapy. J Dermatol 1994;21:308–11.

Ploysangam A, Falciglia GA, Brehm BJ. Effect of marginal zinc deficiency on human growth and development. J Trop Pediatr 1997;43:192-8.

Prasad AS. Zinc deficiency: its characterization and treatment. Met Ions Biol Syst 2004;41:103-37.

Rink L, Gabriel P. Zinc and the immune system. Proc Nutr Soc 2000;59:541-52.

Rothman KJ, Moore LL, Singer MR, et al. Teratogenicity of high vitamin A intake. N Engl J Med. Nov 23 1995;333(21):1369-73.

Rudnicki SA. Prevention and treatment of peripheral neuropathy after bariatric surgery. Curr Treat Options Neurol. 2010 Jan;12(1):29-36.

Russell RM. The vitamin A spectrum: from deficiency to toxicity. Am J Clin Nutr. Apr 2000;71(4):878-84.

Russell RM. Vitamin and trace mineral deficiency and excess. In: Braunwald E, Fauci A, Kasper D, et al, eds. Harrison's Principles of Internal Medicine. vol 1. 15th ed. New York, NY: McGraw-Hill; 2001:465-6.

Scheven, BA & Hamilton, NJ. Retinoic acid and 1,25-dihydroxyvitamin D3 stimulate osteoclast formation by different mechanisms. Bone 1990;11:53–9.

Schwartz, RA. Carotenemia. Medscape eMedicine, 5/27/2011. http://emedicine.medscape.com/article/1104368-overview. accessed 9/2011.

Scopinaro N, Adami GF, Marinari GM, et al. Biliopancreatic diversion. World J Surg 1998;22:936 —46.

Slater GH, Ren CJ, Seigel N, et al. Serum fat-soluble vitamin deciency and abnormal calcium metabolism after malabsorptive bariatric surgery. J Gastrointest Surg 2004;8:48 —55.

Stephens NG, Parsons A, Randomised controlled trial of vitamin E in patients with coronary disease: Cambridge Heart Antioxidant Study (CHAOS). Lancet. Mar 23 1996;347(9004):781-6.

Tagami T, Tamanaha T, Shimazu S, et al. Lipid Profiles in the Untreated Patients with Hashimoto Thyroiditis and the Effects of Thyroxine Treatment on Subclinical Hypothyroidism with Hashimoto Thyroiditis. Endocr J. Dec 22 2009.

Takita Y, Ichimiya M, Hamamoto Y, Muto M. A case of carotenemia associated with ingestion of nutrient supplements. J Dermatol. Feb 2006;33(2):132-4.

Tanyel MC, Mancano LD. Neurologic findings in vitamin E deficiency. Am Fam Physician. Jan 1997;55(1):197-201.

Togari, A, Kondo, M, Arai, M & Matsumoto, S. Effects of retinoic acid on bone formulation and resorption in cultured mouse calvaria. Gen Pharmacol 1991;22:287–92.

Toral GM, Figuerola J, Negro JJ. Multiple ways to become red: Pigment identification in red feathers using spectrometry. Comp Biochem Physiol B Biochem Mol Biol. Mar 4 2008.

Traber MG, Frei B, Vitamin E revisited: do new data validate benefits for chronic disease prevention? Curr Opin Lipidol. Feb 2008;19(1):30-8.

Van Wouwe JP. Clinical and laboratory assessment of zinc deficiency in Dutch children. A review. Biol Trace Elem Res 1995;49:211-25.

Walker J, Kepner A.Wernicke's encephalopathy presenting as acute psychosis after gastric bypass. J Emerg Med. 2009 Apr 28.

Wang LC, Busbey S. Images in clinical medicine. Acquired acrodermatitis enteropathica. N Engl J Med 2005;352:1121.

Wu K, Platz EA, Willett WC, et al. A randomized trial on folic acid supplementation and risk of recurrent colorectal adenoma. Am J Clin Nutr. 2009;90(6):1623-1631.

Yusuf S, Dagenais G, Vitamin E supplementation and cardiovascular events in high-risk patients. The Heart Outcomes Prevention Evaluation Study Investigators. N Engl J Med. Jan 20 2000;342(3):154-60.

Index

Index

NFPA: Making Clinical Connections

Index

Index